How to Use This Saunders Nursing Survival Guide

This book presents need-to-know information on ECGs and the Heart in a complete, easy-to-learn format to help you master one of the most difficult subjects in nursing.

These headings walk you through each chapter:

What You WILL LEARN An introductory list of checkpoints to outline what is covered in each chapter.

What It IS A "short and sweet" section devoted to the definition and description of the topic.

What You NEED TO KNOW The essential information and skills to be mastered, with a discussion of why they are important.

What You DO Nursing interventions that apply everything you learned in the What You NEED TO KNOW section.

Do You UNDERSTAND? Various activities and exercises (with answers) so you can review and make sure you understand each topic.

Technical terms (and common hospital terms) are given easy-to-understand explanations, and if you're likely to hear something referred to in a certain way in the hospital setting, we've highlighted the term in color.

These icons punctuate the text:

 Highlights the most important points to study or use in the clinical atmosphere.

 Alerts you to urgent information about dangerous conditions and how to avoid them.

 Guides you through formulas and problem-solving (with examples).

 Points out age-related variations in signs and symptoms, nursing interventions, and patient teaching.

 Clues you in to possible variations related to a patient's cultural background.

 Instructs you to head to the Internet for additional resources.

Tell Us What YOU Think

The *Saunders Nursing Survival Guide Series* has been created with the help of student feedback to serve your nursing review needs. In order to continue this tradition we invite you to voice your opinion. A website has been created to allow you the opportunity to Tell Us What YOU Think. Please, go to the website SNSGSurvey.elsevier.com, and help us continue to provide you with student focused and friendly review activities. Your ideas will be used to create new and fun ways for students like you to learn and review the difficult topics they face throughout their nursing education.

Go to: SNSGSurvey.elsevier.com and Tell Us What YOU Think.
YOU Think.

Saunders
Nursing Survival Guide
ECGs
& the Heart

SECOND EDITION

Cynthia Chernecky, PhD, RN, CNS, AOCN
Professor, Department of
Physiological and Technological
Nursing
Medical College of Georgia School
of Nursing
Augusta, Georgia

Kitty Garrett, RN, MSN, CCRN
Critical Care Clinical Nurse
Specialist
St. Joseph Hospital
Augusta, Georgia

Beverly George-Gay, RN, MSN, CCRN
Assistant Professor
Department of Nurse Anesthesia
Virginia Commonwealth University
School of Allied Health
Richmond, Virginia

Rebecca K. Hodges, MSN, RN, CCRN
Critical Care Clinical Nurse
Specialist
St. Joseph Hospital
Augusta, Georgia

M. Christine Alichnie, PhD, RN
Chairperson and Professor
Department of Nursing
Assistant Dean
School of Health Sciences
Bloomsburg University
Bloomsburg, Pennsylvania

Cynthia L. Terry, RN, CCRN
Assistant Professor, Nursing Program
LeHigh Carbon Community
College
Schnecksville, Pennsylvania;
Staff Nurse, Intensive Care Unit
Warren Hospital
Phillipsburg, New Jersey

SAUNDERS

ELSEVIER

11830 Westline Industrial Drive
St. Louis, Missouri 63146

Acquisitions Editor: Catherine Jackson
Developmental Editor: Amanda Sunderman Politte
Publishing Services Manager: Jeff Patterson
Designer: Jyotika Shroff

Printed and bound by CPI Group (UK) Ltd, Croydon, CR0 4YY

Transferred to digital print 2012

About the Authors

Dr. Cynthia Chernecky earned her degrees at the University of Connecticut (BSN), the University of Pittsburgh (MN), and Case Western Reserve University (PhD). She also earned an NCI fellowship at Yale University and a postdoctorate visiting scholarship at UCLA. She is the coordinator of the Acute & Critical Care Clinical Nurse Specialist track and an Advanced Oncology Certified Nurse (AOCN) with over 25 years of clinical practice experience. Her clinical area of expertise is critical care oncology, with over 22 book publications including *Laboratory Tests and Diagnostic Procedures* (fourth edition) and *Advanced and Critical Care Oncology Nursing: Managing Primary Complications*. She is a national and international speaker, researcher, and published scholar in cancer nursing as well as the recipient of numerous awards. She is also active in the Orthodox Church and enjoys life with family, friends, colleagues, and a West Highland white terrier.

Kitty Garrett is a Critical Care Clinical Nurse Specialist at St. Joseph Hospital in Augusta, Georgia. She has 27 years of experience teaching basic dysrhythmias; 12-lead ECGs; and BCLS, ACLS, and CCRN Reviews at St. Joseph Hospital and in the community. She is a national and local member and past program chair of the American Association of Critical Care Nurses and is certified through AACN as a CCRN. She is a clinical instructor of junior nursing students at the Medical College of Georgia. She enjoys gardening, walking, playing tennis, and playing with her two granddaughters.

Beverly George-Gay is an Assistant Professor in the Department of Nurse Anesthesia at the Virginia Commonwealth University School of Allied Health in Richmond, Virginia. She completed her MSN degree at the University of Florida in 1991 and began a career in academic nursing at the Medical College of Georgia, School of Nursing, before relocating to Richmond. Beverly has 20 years of acute and critical care nursing experience. She is an active ACLS and BLS instructor and lectures both locally and nationally on critical care topics. Beverly is a proud wife and mother of three children, Reese, Joseph, and Dominique.

Rebecca (Becki) Hodges is a Critical Care Clinical Nurse Specialist at St. Joseph Hospital in Augusta, Georgia. She received her BSN and MSN from the Medical College of Georgia and has maintained CCRN certification for over 20 years. Becki is a charter member and past President of the CSRA chapter of AACN, is a member of Sigma Theta Tau, and has been named to Who's Who in Nursing. She has co-authored other publications, including *Hemodynamic Monitoring* and *Emergency and Critical Care Nursing*. Becki is also an avid gardener (specializing in topiary and herb gardening) and was a past President of the Azalea Garden Club.

Contributors to the First Edition

Mary Ann Cegielsky, MSN, RN
Assistant Professor
Department of Nursing
Bloomsburg University
Bloomsburg, Pennsylvania

Sharon Kribbs, MN, RN
Assistant Chairperson and Assistant Professor
Department of Nursing
Bloomsburg University
Bloomsburg, Pennsylvania

Roseanne LeVan, MSN, RN
Former Instructor
Department of Nursing
Bloomsburg University
Bloomsburg, Pennsylvania

Dorette Sugg Welk, PhD, MSN, RN
Professor
Department of Nursing
Bloomsburg University
Bloomsburg, Pennsylvania

Faculty and Student Reviewers of the First Edition

FACULTY

Betty Nash Blevins, MSN, RN, CCRN, CS
Bluefield State College
Bluefield, West Virginia

Elizabeth M. Christensen, RN, MN, CCRN
Affiliate Faculty
University of Phoenix
New Orleans, Louisiana

Ronald Mitchell, PhD, RN
Idaho State University
Pocatello, Idaho

Jay K. Ober, RN, BS, CCRN, CEN
Cardiac Intensive Care Unit
Baystate Medical Center
Springfield, Massachusetts

Elizabeth A. O'Connor, MSN, RN, CS, FNP, CCRN
Bozeman College of Nursing
Montana State University, Great Falls Campus
Bozeman, Montana

Thena E. Parrott, PhD, RNCS
Associate Degree Nursing Program
Blinn College
Bryan, Texas

Jeffrey J. Paurus, RN, MS
Instructor
Minneapolis Community and Technical College
Staff Nurse
Fairview University Hospital
Minneapolis, Minnesota

Nancy L. Sarpy, RN, MS, CCRN
Assistant Professor of Nursing
School of Nursing
Loma Linda University
Loma Linda, California

STUDENTS

Edith Benham, LPN
WorWic Community College
Salisbury, Maryland

Kimberly A. Bloom
Bloomsburg University
Bloomsburg, Pennsylvania

Evelyn DeMoss
Austin Community College
Austin, Texas

Christine Griffin
Child Care Counselor
Lehigh Carbon Community College
Schnecksville, Pennsylvania

Elizabeth Hartzell, CNA
Lehigh Carbon Community College
Schnecksville, Pennsylvania

Carol A. Haverty, CAN
Lehigh Carbon Community College
Schnecksville, Pennsylvania

Sheila Holliday
Austin Community College
Austin, Texas

Mary Jo Lampart
Bloomsburg University
Bloomsburg, Pennsylvania

Nicole E. Landis
Lehigh Carbon Community College
Schnecksville, Pennsylvania

John Daniel Luchansky
Bloomsburg University
Bloomsburg, Pennsylvania

Maria E. Mulinos, LPN
Nanticoke Memorial Hospital
Seaford, Delaware

Melissa L. Normann
Bloomsburg University
Bloomsburg, Pennsylvania

Michelle Ratliff, CNA
Lehigh Carbon Community College
Schnecksville, Pennsylvania

Frederic W. Strohl, LPN
President, Phi Theta Kappa
Presidential Ambassador, SGA Senator
Lehigh Carbon Community College
Schnecksville, Pennsylvania

Dina M. Timko
Bloomsburg University
Bloomsburg, Pennsylvania

Deborah Warner, CNA
Lehigh Carbon Community College
Schnecksville, Pennsylvania

Beata F. Wirth
President, Student Nurse Program
College Senator, Phi Theta Kappa
Lehigh Carbon Community College
Schnecksville, Pennsylvania

Series Reviewers

FACULTY

Edwina A. McConnell, PhD, RN, FRCNA
Professor
School of Nursing
Texas Technical University Health Sciences Center
Lubbock, Texas
Consultant
Gorham, Maine

Judith L, Myers, MSN, RN
Health Sciences Center
St. Louis University School of Nursing
St. Louis, Missouri

STUDENTS

Joy Kutlenios Amos, RN, BSN
Piedmont Medical Center
Rock Hill, South Carolina;
Former student
Wheeling Jesuit University
Wheeling, West Virginia

Angela M. Boyd, AS
University of Tennessee at Martin
Martin, Tennessee

Shayne Michael Gray, RN, BSN
University of Arkansas
Little Rock, Arkansas

Jill Hall, RN
Miller Children's Hospital
Long Beach, California

Jennifer Hamilton
University of Virginia
Charlottesville, Virginia

Elizabeth J. Hoogmoed, RN, BSN
Valley Hospital
Ridgewood, New Jersey

Katie Scarlett McRae, BA, BSN
Oregon Health Sciences University
Portland, Oregon

Preface

The *Saunders Nursing Survival Guide* series was created with your input. Nursing students told us about the topics they found more difficult to master, such as fluids and electrolytes, drug calculations, ECGs, pathophysiology, and pharmacology. Focus groups were held at the National Student Nurses Association meeting, and we asked you what the best way would be to learn this difficult material. Your responses were certainly interesting! You said we should keep the text to a minimum; use an engaging, fun approach; provide ample space to write on the pages; include a variety of activities to appeal to students with different learning styles; make the content visually appealing; and provide NCLEX review questions so you could check your understanding of key topics and perform any necessary review. The *Saunders Nursing Survival Guide* series is the result of your ideas.

An understanding of the heart and its electrical conduction system is necessary for excellence in nursing care, and an ability to apply knowledge related to the heart is also needed throughout the nursing process. Such knowledge provides an avenue for nursing assessment, leading to an increased quality and quantity of life for all those for whom nurses care.

Such knowledge is also the focus of *ECGs & the Heart.* To understand the diagnostic ECG test associated with the heart, you need to comprehend the electrophysiology of the heart muscle. You then need to incorporate knowledge of ECG leads to their specific cardiac areas and learn to interpret their output, which provides guidelines for care and intervention. We have made every effort to discuss similar principles of ECG interpretation as a related group of concepts to help you understand ECG interpretation and its relationship to cardiac electrophysiology. However, ECG output is only one diagnostic test and one piece of assessment datum. You must examine the entire picture of a patient before interventions are implemented, and this book will help you understand the heart muscle, how the conduction system works, and how to incorporate ECG data into your larger plan of care.

We include many features in the margins to help you focus on the vital information you'll need to succeed in the classroom and in the clinical setting:

- **TAKE HOME POINTS** are composed of both study tips for classroom tests and "pearls of wisdom" to assist you in caring for patients. Both are drawn from our many years of combined academic and clinical experience.
- Content marked with a **CAUTION** icon ▼ is vital and usually involves nursing actions that may have life-threatening consequences or significantly affect patient outcomes.
- The **LIFESPAN** icon 🐢 and the **CULTURE** icon ☯ highlight variations in treatment that may be necessary for specific age or ethnic groups.
- A **CALCULTOR** icon 📱 will draw your eye to important equations and examples that will help you calculate proper medication dosages.
- A **WEB LINKS** icon 🖥 will direct you to sites on the Internet that give more detailed information on a given topic.

Each of these icons specifically helps you focus on real-world patient care, the nursing process, and positive patient outcomes.

We also use consistent headings that emphasize specific nursing actions.

- **What You WILL LEARN** provides a list of the concepts to be learned in that chapter.
- **What It IS** provides a definition of a topic.
- **What You NEED TO KNOW** provides the explanation of the topic.
- **What You DO** explains what you do as a practicing nurse.
- **Do You UNDERSTAND** provides questions and exercises that are both appropriate and useful to reinforce the topic's concepts.

This five-step approach provides you with information and helps you learn how to apply it to the clinical setting.

We have used our own clinical experiences, our memories of being nursing students, and the expert experiences of nursing faculty, clinicians, and current nursing students to bring you a text that will help you understand ECGs and the heart and therefore implement better patient care. We believe that understanding is the key to critical thinking and that critical thinking is the key to the art and science of nursing.

We believe that this book and this series will result in excellent nursing care. The desire to acquire knowledge is never-ending, so let us begin the quest with *ECG's & the Heart!*

Cynthia Chernecky, PhD, RN, CNS, AOCN
Kitty Garrett, RN, MSN, CCRN
Beverly George-Gay, RN, MSN, CCRN
Rebecca K. Hodges, MSN, RN, CCRN

Acknowledgments

This edition is packed with clinical expertise and the professionalism of teaching scholars. I want to thank my coeditors for their spirit of teamwork and their dedication to making health care more advanced. This book has been a labor of love for all of us and you need extraordinary persons to realize such an outcome of excellence. Special heartfelt thanks to Becki, Bev, and Kitty for truly caring about patients and students. Your unselfishness and giving spirits have made this book a premier model of caring for persons with ECG changes. I am truly blessed to have all of you as friends as well as professional colleagues

My thanks to the team at Elsevier who has worked with us to produce excellence throughout the production and printing of this book.

To all those who have supported me in realizing that in caring for humanity we truly help our souls, my thanks to my mother Olga Chernecky-McGuinness; Godmother Helen Prohorik; Mother Thecla (Abbess), Mother Helena, and Mother Seraphima of Saints Mary and Martha Orthodox Monastery; nieces Ellie Chernecky and Annie Chernecky; nephew Michael Chernecky; brother Dr. Richard Chernecky; Dr. Ann Kolanowski; Dr. Rich Haas; Dr. Linda Sarna; Dr. Jean Brown; Dr. Leda Danao; Dr. Mary Cooley; Dr. Geri Padilla; Dr. Kathy Wren; Tim Wren; Pat Revolinski; Rebecca Rule; Nancy Stark; Kim Black; and Denise Macklin. To the undergraduate students who make my life challenging and rewarding, I thank you for all your questions and willingness to learn.

Dr. Cynthia (Cinda) Chernecky

Thanks to my husband Michael and to my three sons, Trey, Brian, and Michael, for their patience, understanding, and support during the preparation of this second edition. I would also like to thank Becki Hodges, my partner, coauthor, and friend, who was always there to consult when the need arose. Special thanks to Cinda and Beverly, my faculty mentors, whose gentle persuasion inspired me to contribute to this book. The Elsevier staff has been a pleasure to work with; their patience with the authors is much appreciated.

Kitty Garrett

I would like to acknowledge Cinda Chernecky for being a constant source of inspiration for me. To Kitty and Becki, with whom I truly enjoy working. To my students and colleagues who see the value of lifelong learning. To everyone at Elsevier who has worked on this book, especially Amanda Politte, who keeps us on track. Most importantly to my husband and best friend Mantovani, who supports me in everything I do.

Beverly George-Gay

It is with deep appreciation that I acknowledge those who have brought me endless joy and led me to the path of learning. Thanks to the contributors of this book, who shared their knowledge and made this a reality, and to Amanda Politte and Jeff Patterson at Elsevier. Thanks to Dr. Cinda Chernecky, my mentor, who got me involved in this project. In memory of my dad, Dr. Hubert King, and special thanks to my mom, Betty, who have continually encouraged me and always provided love and support. To Drs. Hurley Jones and Wade Strickland, who first introduced me to the joys of cardiology. I am forever indebted to Kitty Garrett, a coauthor and special friend who was always there for moral support. Finally, the most special thanks to my husband, Jack; my family, Stuart, Paige, Brad, Havird, Hodges, Phyllis, Rob, Riah, Blake, and Jordan; and my sister, Debbie, for their limitless love.

Rebecca Hodges

Contents

Anatomy and Physiology

What You WILL LEARN

After reading this chapter, you will know how to do the following:
- ✔ Name the components of cardiac output.
- ✔ Describe the pathway of circulation through the heart.
- ✔ Trace the conduction system through the heart.
- ✔ Name the three main branches of the coronary arteries.

What IS the Heart?

The *heart* is a muscular organ that is about the size of a fist, and is located between the second and sixth left ribs and behind the sternum.

It is composed of four chambers: two *atria* and two *ventricles*. The main function of the atria, located at the top of the heart, is to act as reservoirs for incoming blood. However, the atria also contribute as much as 30% to the output of blood from the heart. This output of blood from the atria is known as *atrial kick*.

The ventricles are the heart's main pumping chambers. They are separated by valves that promote forward flow and allow synchrony between the filling and pumping of blood. The valves between the atria and ventricles are called the *atrioventricular* (AV) *valves*. These include the *tricuspid valve* and the *mitral valve*. The tricuspid valve separates the right atrium from the right ventricle, and the mitral valve separates the left atrium from the left ventricle.

The valves leading away from the heart are called the *semilunar valves*. These include the *aortic valve* and the *pulmonic valve*. The aortic valve separates the left ventricle from the aorta, and the pulmonic valve separates the right ventricle from the pulmonary artery. To be competent, valves must open and close easily.

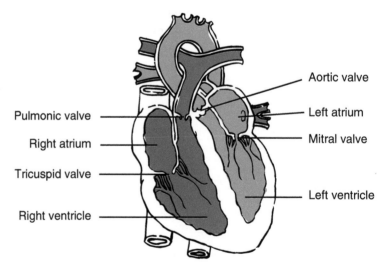

Redrawn from Guyton, Hall: *Textbook of medical physiology,* ed 10, Philadelphia, 2000, Saunders.

The heart has four layers: (1) the *myocardium,* (2) the *endocardium,* (3) the *epicardium,* and (4) the *pericardium.* The myocardium is the main muscular layer. This is the layer that is injured in a *myocardial infarction* (MI). The endocardium is the inner lining, which is continuous with the valves and the *endothelium* that lines the blood vessels. The epicardium is the outer surface from which the coronary arteries originate. The pericardium is a fibrous sac that surrounds and protects the heart.

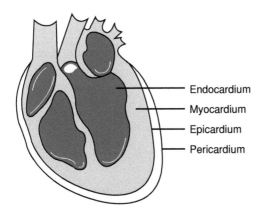

— Endocardium
— Myocardium
— Epicardium
— Pericardium

American Heart Association
www.americanheart.org

Heart sounds are caused by the closure of valves. The first heart sound (lub), or S1, is caused by closure of the AV valves. The second heart sound (dup), or S2, is caused by closure of the semilunar valves. A valve that does not close tightly allows backflow of blood (i.e., **insufficiency** or **regurgitation**). A valve that does not open wide enough causes turbulent flow secondary to obstruction or narrowing (i.e., **stenosis**). Both of these conditions may be detected clinically by auscultating for a murmur specific to the valve involved.

TAKE HOME POINTS
- Subendocardium is used to describe the portion of the myocardium that is closest to the inner lining of the heart, but does not go through the entire thickness of the heart muscle.
- *Transmural* refers to the full thickness of the myocardium.

What You NEED TO KNOW

There are three systems that must work together for the heart to beat efficiently: (1) circulatory, (2) conduction, and (3) coronary. The circulatory system is the continuous network of vessels through which the heart mechanically pumps blood. The conduction system is the electrical wiring system that stimulates the heart to pump. The coronary system is a system of arteries and veins that provide oxygenated blood to meet the metabolic needs of the heart muscle itself. The heart has two types of cells. Myocardial cells have contractile units that allow the cell to contract when the cell is electrically stimulated. Pacemaker cells are specialized cells that can spontaneously generate and conduct electrical impulses.

Circulatory System

The heart is actually two pumps in one. The left side pumps blood through the arterial system to deliver oxygenated blood to the tissues; the right side receives blood returning from the body and pumps it to the lungs to be reoxygenated. Although the left and right sides of the heart are separated by a septum, they pump in synchrony with each other. While the left ventricle is ejecting blood to the aorta, the right ventricle is ejecting blood to the pulmonary artery and out to the lungs.

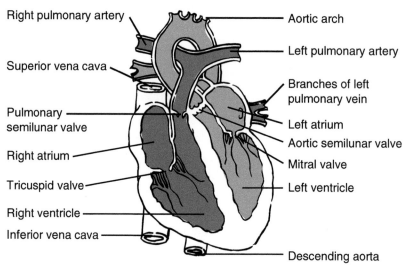

Redrawn from Thibodeau, Patton: *Anatomy & physiology, St Louis, 1987, Mosby, as presented in McCance, Huether: Pathophysiology: the biologic basis for disease in adults & children, ed 3, St Louis, 1998, Mosby, p. 971.*

The right heart receives venous blood from the systemic circulation through the *superior* and *inferior vena cavae,* which enter the right atrium. Blood leaves the right ventricle and enters the pulmonary circulation through the pulmonary artery. The pulmonary artery divides into right and left pulmonary arteries to transport nonoxygenated blood from the right heart to the right and left lungs.

The pulmonary arteries branch further into the pulmonary capillary bed, where oxygen and carbon dioxide exchange occurs. The four pulmonary veins, two from the right lung and two from the left lung, carry oxygenated blood from the lungs to the left side of the heart. The oxygenated blood moves through the left atrium and ventricle and out into the aorta, which delivers the blood to systemic arteries and arterioles that supply the body.

The left ventricular muscle is thicker than the right because it has to work harder to generate higher pressures to pump blood throughout the body. The right ventricle only has to pump from the heart to the lungs and therefore the wall is thinner.

Each cardiac cycle includes a pumping and resting (*systole* and *diastole*) action. In **systole,** the ventricles contract, the semilunar valves (pulmonic and aortic) open, and the AV valves (mitral and tricuspid) close. Then, during **diastole,** the ventricles refill again from the atria. The AV valves are open, and the semilunar valves are closed. One cycle of filling and contracting is equal to one heartbeat.

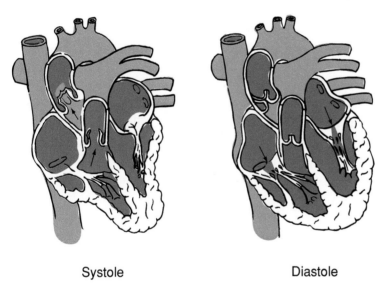

Systole   Diastole

Redrawn from Thibodeau, Patton: *Anatomy & physiology,* St Louis, 1987, Mosby, as presented in McCance, Huether: *Pathophysiology: the biologic basis for disease in adults & children,* ed 3, St Louis, 1998, Mosby, p. 974.

 TAKE HOME POINTS

Ventricular filling occurs during diastole. There are four factors that affect how much blood is pumped from the heart **(cardiac output)** every minute:
1. Heart rate
2. Volume of blood (preload)
3. Amount of resistance (afterload)
4. Squeezing ability of the ventricular myocardium (contractility)

Factors affecting contractility are called *inotropic agents.* Positive inotropic drugs (e.g., digitalis, dobutamine) increase myocardial contractility. Negative inotropic drugs (e.g., β-blockers, calcium channel blockers) decrease myocardial contractility.

Cardiac Output

Cardiac output is the amount of blood pumped out of the heart every minute. It is determined by the heart rate and the stroke volume. If cardiac output is compromised, oxygen delivery to the tissues of the body will decrease. The heart rate should not be too fast or too slow. If it is too slow, there is not enough stimulation to pump enough blood out. If it is too fast, there is not enough time for the ventricles to fill in between beats. Either way, the amount of blood pumped out to the body can be compromised.

The stroke volume is the amount of blood pumped out of the heart with each heartbeat. It is determined by three factors—preload, afterload, and contractility. The heart must have enough blood volume to fill and stretch the left ventricle to maximize its contraction, but not so much that the ventricle is overstretched and unable to keep up with the demand. The stretching caused by blood in the left ventricle is called *preload.* Remember the Frank-Starling curve: "The greater the stretch, the more forceful the contraction—up to a point."

The heart also needs to pump freely without meeting excessive resistance. The main cause of resistance is constriction of the blood vessels *(arterioles).* This constriction increases the aortic pressure and causes the heart to work harder to get the blood through the constricted vessels. This is called *afterload.*

Finally, the squeezing ability of the ventricular myocardium affects the amount of blood pumped from the heart. The force of the contraction depends on the degree of fiber shortening (**contractility**). Two major factors determine the force of contraction: (1) **preload** and (2) **sympathetic nervous system stimulation.** Stimulation of the sympathetic nervous system increases myocardial contractility. If the muscle fibers are not well-oxygenated or if they have been damaged by past heart attacks, over-stretching of fibers, depressant effects of drugs, or electrolyte imbalances, myocardial fibers may not shorten maximally.

Conduction System

How is the heart stimulated to beat? The heart's own internal pacemaker, called the **sinoatrial** (SA) **node,** stimulates the heart to beat. The SA node is a specialized bundle of nerve fibers located at the junction of the superior vena cava and right atrium, near the epicardial surface. The SA node "fires" by a process called depolarization. Depolarization occurs when the inside of the cell becomes more positive due to the movement of sodium and potassium ions. Then the heart must rest before it starts over again; this process is called repolarization. Repolarization occurs when sodium and potassium move back to their starting positions, allowing the cell to return to a negative resting state.

The firing of the SA node stimulates both the right and the left atria (atrial depolarization) and causes them to contract. The impulse then travels through a network of three internodal tracts that connect the SA node to the *atrioventricular* (AV) *node.* The AV node, also known as the *AV junction,* is located in the inferior portion of the right atrial wall, directly above the right ventricle. Once the impulse has reached the AV node, it is delayed for a short time to allow the ventricles to fill. It then continues from the AV node down a common pathway called the *bundle of His* and splits into two branches (the left and right bundle branches). These lead to the left and right ventricles, respectively.

The left bundle branch further divides into an anterior and posterior branch. The terminal portions of the bundle branches are called *Purkinje fibers*. The Purkinje fibers are like small fingers that reach throughout the myocardium to stimulate the ventricular muscle. This electrical activation of the muscle cells is called *ventricular depolarization*. Ventricular depolarization initiates ventricular contraction. After depolarization, the cells are then deactivated—a process called *ventricular repolarization*. There is no physical response to repolarization. It is just an electrical phenomenon. The cycle is then repeated for each heart beat.

During ventricular repolarization, while the cells are trying to get back to normal, they are unable to respond to another stimulus. This is called the "refractory period." In early repolarization, the "absolute refractory period" is a time when the myocardial cells will not respond to *any* stimulation. But then there is a brief (millisecond) period called the "relative refractory period" when ventricular cells may respond if a strong enough stimulus comes along. The cells will depolarize out of synchrony, causing dysrhythmias. For this reason, ventricular repolarization is often called the "vulnerable period."

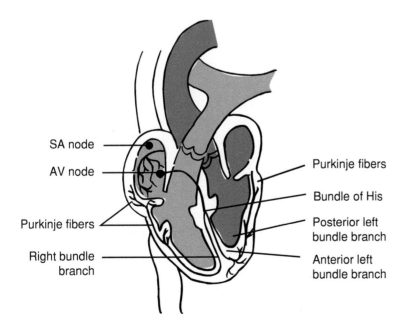

SA node

AV node

Purkinje fibers

Right bundle branch

Purkinje fibers

Bundle of His

Posterior left bundle branch

Anterior left bundle branch

⚠️ If the heart beats too slowly, tissue oxygenation is affected. Also, if the heart beats too rapidly, there is less time between beats for the ventricles to fill. This can cause a decrease in the amount of blood pumped from the heart, which can also decrease tissue perfusion.

🏠 TAKE HOME POINTS

- The electrical energy produced by the movement of the sodium and potassium ions is what stimulates the heart to beat.
- It is imperative to be familiar with the conduction system to understand normal and abnormal heart rhythms (dysrhythmias).

Cardiac cells are unique in several ways. The ability of the heart to conduct impulses by stimulating adjacent cells located along a pathway is called "conductivity." The ability of the cell to shorten, resulting in cardiac muscle contraction is called "contractility."

The property of "automaticity" is what allows the SA node to initiate an impulse on its own. It does not need stimulation from the nervous system to do so. All pacemaker cells have this ability, but it is enhanced in the SA node. Although the SA node is the "normal" pacemaker of the heart, certain characteristics of cardiac cells allow them to occasionally interfere with the rhythm of the heart. Cells outside of the conduction system can exhibit automaticity and initiate an impulse on their own. The property of "excitability" allows the cell to respond to the stimulus, and then conduct it to other cells to cause a contraction. Thus, if a cell in the atria, the AV node, or the ventricle decides to fire, it can do so, causing a dysrhythmia. A heartbeat that is initiated anywhere other than the SA node is called an "ectopic" beat.

How does the heart know how fast to beat? The average heart rate is 60 to 100 beats per minute (bpm). Heart rate is determined by a balance of sympathetic and parasympathetic innervation. The normal physiologic response is for the heart rate to change to meet the demands of the body. For example, during exercise the skeletal muscles need more oxygen, and therefore heart rate increases to send more blood to the muscles. However, during sleep metabolic needs are decreased, and therefore heart rate is also decreased. (As a health care provider, you should be prepared to see some of your patients' heart rates drop into the 50s during the night.) In most cases the sympathetic and parasympathetic nervous systems are balanced to keep the heart rate within normal limits. However, one can override the other when it becomes necessary.

Should the SA node fail to fire or fire too slowly, or if the impulse does not make it through to the AV node, the AV node can initiate impulses. The inherent rate of the AV node as the pacemaker is 40 to 60 bpm. If the SA node and the AV node fail to fire, fire too slowly, or the impulse fails to reach the ventricles, the ventricles can also stimulate themselves from the Purkinje fibers. However, this is the least efficient "pacemaker," because the ventricles can only initiate impulses at a rate of 20 to 40 bpm. This rate is too slow to meet the body's oxygenation needs, and the patient will require an artificial pacemaker to maintain cardiac output. These rhythms, which arise from the AV node or ventricles, are protective in nature and arise out of necessity rather than irritability. They are called "escape rhythms."

Coronary Circulation

The heart beats an average of 70 times a minute, 24 hours a day, 7 days a week for a lifetime. Unlike other body organs, it never gets a break. The heart has its own circulatory system to supply the myocardium with the necessary blood and oxygen. The heart "feeds itself first." It pumps an average of 5 to 6 L of blood every minute. The system of blood vessels supplying the heart is called the *coronary system.* The left and right coronary arteries branch off of the aorta just past the aortic valve. Most coronary filling occurs during diastole.

The left coronary artery descends in a common branch called the *left main* and then divides into the *left anterior descending* (LAD) and *circumflex arteries.* The LAD feeds the interventricular septum and anterior left ventricle. The circumflex feeds the left atrium and the lateral portion of the left ventricle.

The right coronary artery descends and winds around the back of the heart. It feeds the right atrium, the SA and AV nodes, the right ventricle, and the inferior and posterior surfaces of the left ventricle.

TAKE HOME POINTS

Ectopic beats
Although the SA node is the *normal pacemaker* of the heart, every cell in the heart has the ability to initiate an electrical impulse. The cardiac properties of automaticity, excitability, and conductivity explain how ectopic beats and rhythms can form. Common triggers for ectopic beats are ischemia, hypoxemia, electrolyte imbalances, caffeine, nicotine, and emotional stress.

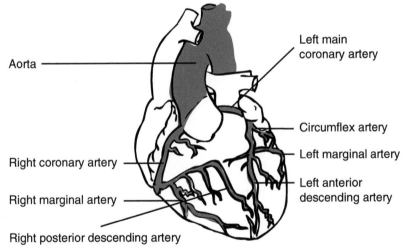

Left main coronary artery

Aorta

Circumflex artery

Left marginal artery

Right coronary artery

Left anterior descending artery

Right marginal artery

Right posterior descending artery

Redrawn from Thibodeau, Patton: *Anatomy & physiology,* St Louis, 1987, Mosby, as presented in McCance, Huether: *Pathophysiology: the biologic basis for disease in adults & children,* ed 3, St Louis, 1998, Mosby, p. 977.

The coronary arteries may develop *atherosclerosis.* Atherosclerotic plaque narrows the lumen of the blood vessels, thereby compromising the blood flow to the myocardium. This can lead to ischemia, causing angina and, ultimately, MI.

TAKE HOME POINTS
The coronary arteries originate on the epicardial surface of the myocardium and terminate on the endocardial surface, which explains why subendocardial ischemia, or ST depression, is the earliest ECG sign of ischemia. A strong knowledge of coronary artery anatomy is needed to interpret ECG results and to locate MI.

Do You UNDERSTAND?

DIRECTIONS: **Complete the crossword puzzle.**

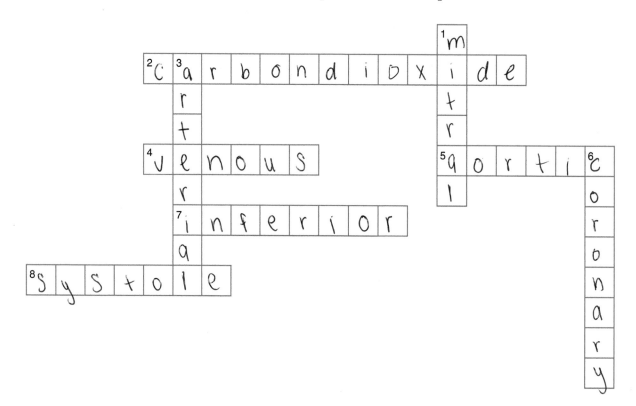

Across

2. The major gaseous waste product from heart circulation.
4. Blood is collected back to the heart by the _____ system.
5. This valve is located between the left ventricle and aorta, and it produces the S2 sound when closing.
7. The bottom of the heart is called the _____ surface.
8. Ventricular contraction.

Down

1. This valve is located between the left atrium and left ventricle and produces the S1 sound when closing.
3. Blood is pumped to the body through the _____ system.
6. These arteries supply the heart with oxygenated blood.

Answers:

DIRECTIONS: **Match column A with the terms listed in column B.**

	Column A	Column B
1. B	Resistance the heart pumps against	a. Preload
2. D	Number of heartbeats per minute	b. Afterload
3. A	Volume and stretch of the heart	c. Contractility
4. C	Squeezing ability of the heart	d. Heart rate

DIRECTIONS: **Place the following electrical events in chronologic order.**
1. _4_ ventricular depolarization
2. _2_ atrial repolarization
3. _1_ ventricular repolarization
4. _3_ atrial depolarization

DIRECTIONS: **Match the following properties of cardiac cells with their definitions**

1. B	ability to respond to an impulse	a. conductivity
2. C	ability to shorten heart fibers to squeeze blood out	b. excitability
3. D	ability to initiate an impulse spontaneously	c. contractility
4. A	ability to spread the impulse to surrounding cells	d. automaticity

DIRECTIONS: **Indicate whether the following statement is <u>true</u> or false.**

Most abnormal heart rhythms are dangerous if they are too fast, too slow, or asynchronous.

Answer: True.
Answers: 1. b; 2. c; 3. d; 4. a.
Answers: 4, 2, 1, 3.
Answers: 1. b; 2. d; 3. a; 4. c.

DIRECTIONS: Label the parts of the conduction system:

a. _____

b. _____

c. _____

d. _____

c. _____

e. _____

f. _____

g. _____

References

AACN Ask the Expert, Posting Waveform Tracing Strips. Last Updated May, 2003. www.aacn.org/aacn/practice.nsf. Then click on "Short Titles", 18(6).

Aehlert B: *ECGs made easy*, ed 2, St Louis, 2002, Mosby.

Alspach JG: *AACN core curriculum for critical care nursing*, ed 5, Philadelphia, 1998, Saunders.

American Heart Association: *Advanced cardiac life support provider manual*, Dallas, 1997, American Heart Association.

Lamborn ML, Moseley MJ: Cardiac alterations. In Hartshorn JC, Sole ML, Lamborn ML, editors: *Introduction to critical care nursing*, ed 3, Philadelphia, 2001, Saunders.

McCance KL: Structure & function of the cardiovascular & lymphatic systems. In McCance KL, Huether SE, editors: *Pathophysiology: the biologic basis for disease in adults and children*, ed 3, St Louis, 1998, Mosby.

Stewart SL, Vitello-Ciccio JM: Cardiovascular clinical physiology. In Kinney et al, editors: *AACN clinical reference for critical care nursing*, ed 4, St Louis, 1998, Mosby.

Answers: a. SA node; b. AV node; c. Purkinje fibers; d. right bundle branch; e. bundle of His; f. posterior left bundle branch; g. anterior left bundle branch.

NCLEX® Review

1. Which chamber of the heart pumps oxygenated blood back into the circulatory system?
   1 Right atrium
   2 Right ventricle
   3 Mitral valve
   4 Left ventricle

2. Another name for ventricular contraction is:
   1 Systole
   2 Diastole
   3 Cyanosis
   4 Sternum

3. The electrical power source of the heart is the SA node. It is located in the:
   1 Right ventricle
   2 Right atrium
   3 Aorta
   4 Left atrium

4. Which of the following medications does not have a positive inotropic effect on the myocardium?
   1 Dobutamine
   2 Digitalis
   3 Propranolol
   4 Epinephrine

5. Another name for the volume of blood in the ventricle immediately before it is ejected is
   1 Preload
   2 Afterload
   3 Contractility
   4 Cardiac index

NCLEX® Review Answers

1. 4 The left ventricle pumps blood into the systemic circulation. The right atrium pumps blood to the right ventricle. The mitral valve is not a heart chamber. The right ventricle pumps blood to the lungs.

2. 1 Systole is ventricular contraction. Diastole is ventricular filling. Cyanosis is a bluish tint to the skin and oral mucosa because of a lack of oxygen. The sternum is the breast bone.

3. 2 The sinoatrial node is located in the right atrium. The right ventricle leads to the pulmonary artery. The aorta is the main blood vessel leading to the body. The left atrium is the heart chamber that receives oxygenated blood from the lungs.

4. 3 Propranolol has a negative inotropic effect on the myocardium (decreasing cardiac contractility). Dobutamine, digitalis, and epinephrine are positive inotropic drugs.

5. 1 The correct answer is preload. Afterload is the resistance that the LV must pump against. Contractility is the squeezing ability of the LV. Cardiac index is cardiac output corrected to body size.

Notes

Chapter 2

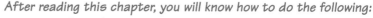

Reference Points for Rhythm Strip Measurements

What You WILL LEARN

After reading this chapter, you will know how to do the following:
- ✔ Define voltage.
- ✔ Describe measuring time.
- ✔ State what should be documented regarding time and voltage.

Electrocardiograms (ECGs) provide information about time and voltage of electrical events in the heart. To obtain these measurements, you need to understand important reference points on the ECG recording paper. This chapter is focused on how to measure *time and voltage* on ECG paper.

What IS Measuring Time and Voltage?

The ECG is printed on ruled paper with vertical and horizontal lines. These lines make up small boxes with thin lines, inside large boxes with heavy lines. Each small box is 1 mm in height and 1 mm in length. Each large box contains 25 small boxes. Height indicates voltage on the vertical axis, measured in millimeters (mm) or millivolts (mV). Width indicates time on the horizontal axis, measured in seconds.

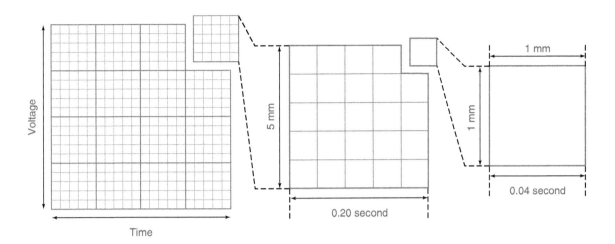

Both time and voltage are measured from the baseline. It is important to view this as an imaginary line drawn through the ECG complex, starting from the beginning of the P wave and continuing on the paper to the end of the T waveform. The height and depth of a wave produced when taking an ECG is measured from the baseline. The baseline is the flat portion of the ECG tracing when there are neither upward nor downward waves (deflections). When you record a strip, the ECG tracing must be flat (not moving up and down) across the page as in the following example. If the tracing is not flat, you will need to troubleshoot the equipment and check your patient. (See Chapter 6 for more information about troubleshooting ECG waveforms.)

Baseline

TAKE HOME POINTS

- The large boxes on ECG paper are identified by heavy black lines.
- To measure time, count the number of small boxes across the horizontal line.
- Multiply the number of small boxes within a wave form by 0.04 seconds (5 × 0.04 = 0.20 seconds) to get the time duration of the wave.
- Five large boxes (or 25 small boxes) on the horizontal line equal 1 second.
- Identify whether you have 1, 3, or 6 second markers on your ECG recording paper.

What You NEED TO KNOW

Measuring Time

One of the main goals of obtaining an ECG is to determine the patient's heart rate and its regularity. Therefore the ECG recording paper must be able to measure time. Time can be measured by counting the small and large boxes on the horizontal axis of the ECG paper, or it can be measured by the *second markers* (small, regularly spaced marks at the top or bottom of the ECG paper). As a health care provider, you should be familiar with both of these time-measurement methods.

Measuring time by counting boxes. Time can be measured by counting the number of boxes that encompass each waveform along the horizontal axis of the ECG paper.

Each small box on a horizontal line is equal to 0.04 seconds (or 40 milliseconds [ms]), and five small boxes on a horizontal line equal one large box. Five times 0.04 equals 0.20 seconds. Therefore one large box (measured horizontally) equals 0.20 seconds or 200 ms. Five large boxes equal 1 second.

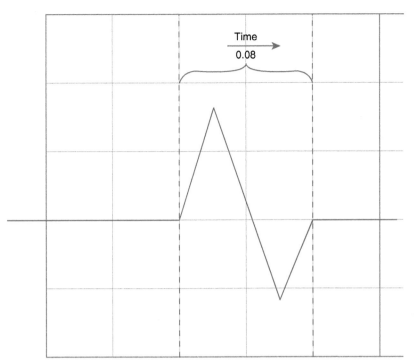

The time duration of each wave of the ECG can be measured by counting the small boxes within a wave on the horizontal line.

Measuring time by second markers. *Second markers* can appear on ECG paper as vertical lines, triangles, or dots (depending on the paper manufacturer). These markers may also be called **tics** or **hatch marks,** and they can occur every 1, 3, or 6 seconds. Second markers are most common in the form of vertical lines.

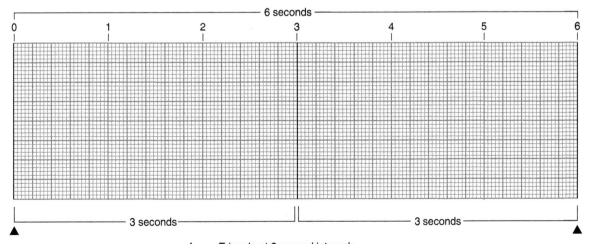

▲ = Triangle at 6-second intervals

| = Hatch mark at 1-second intervals

Remember, five large boxes equal 1 second. This means the marker occurring after every fifth large box indicates a 1-second interval (1 marker per second), a marker after every 15th large box indicates a 3-second interval, and a marker after each 30th large box indicates a 6-second interval.

Most ECG paper has 3- or 6-second markers or both. Because you will analyze and document 6-second strips, it is important to recognize when these markers appear on the ECG paper.

Measuring Voltage

Voltage is measured on the vertical axis. Therefore the height, or depth, of a wave represents a measure of voltage. Voltage is measured either upward or downward from the *isoelectric line.*

Each small vertical box is equal to 0.1 mV. Therefore 10 small vertical boxes or 2 large vertical boxes equal 1 mV. If the heart contracts forcefully or if the patient is experiencing enlargement of the heart muscle (**hypertrophy**), voltage will be increased. This can be observed as increased height (number of vertical boxes) of the waveforms.

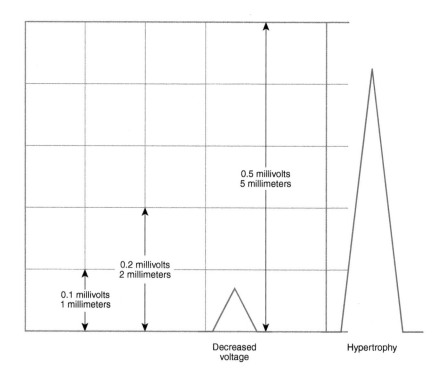

0.5 millivolts
5 millimeters

0.2 millivolts
2 millimeters

0.1 millivolts
1 millimeters

Decreased
voltage

Hypertrophy

If something interferes with heart energy, causing the heart to contract less forcefully (as in *cardiac tamponade*), voltage will be decreased. This will be indicated by decreased height of the waveforms.

Voltage is more closely assessed with the analysis of a 12-lead ECG. For a patient's heartbeat to be counted by a monitor, the voltage of the main, tall waveform needs to be at least 5 mm.

In the clinical setting, voltage is measured in millimeters, not millivolts. For example, when describing the height of an R wave, it is more correct to say that the R wave is 4 mm tall, not 0.04 mV.

TAKE HOME POINTS

Energy (voltage) of the heartbeat is measured up and down on the ECG paper. Each small box (up or down) is 0.1 mV, or 1.0 mm. Each large box (up or down) is 0.5 mV, or 5 mm.

What You DO

Measuring different waveforms and intervals across time in the cardiac cycle requires you to measure distances across the horizontal line.

• To measure time accurately, use ECG calipers.

Redrawn from Sole, Hartshorn, Lamborn: *Introduction to critical care nursing,* ed 3, Philadelphia, 2001, Saunders, p. 52.

• Hold the calipers in your dominant hand, with your thumb over the upper-middle-front section and your index finger just behind the back of the calipers.
• Use your middle finger to prevent the two tips from slipping. This technique is not unlike holding a pencil when writing.

To measure from point A to point B on the following rhythm strip:

Lead II   A   BC

- Place the left tip of your caliper on point A and the right tip of your caliper on point B. Remember, measurements are always done on the baseline.
- Do not try to count the number of boxes between the calipers from these two points. Instead, hold your calipers to prevent movement.
- Without changing the width of the caliper tips, raise them from the ECG tracing to an area of the graph paper where there is a clear view of the horizontal lines.

There should be four small boxes from A to B. This indicates that 0.16 seconds (4 × 0.04 = 0.16) passed during this area of electrical stimulation. On the same strip, look at the parts labeled B and C.

- Place the left tip of your caliper on point B and the right tip on point C.
- Carefully lift the caliper to the top of the graphics without changing the distance between caliper tips.
- Count the number of boxes between the two tips.

There should be two small boxes between B and C. This indicates that it took 0.08 seconds for this wave of stimulation to travel down the conduction system of the heart.

To measure an ECG rhythm strip without calipers:

- Take a clean piece of paper and line it up under the baseline of the cardiac cycle you are measuring.
- Place a small vertical mark on the beginning of the waveform that you want to measure (on the left) and another at the end of the waveform (on the right).
- Place the paper at the top of the graphic area, and count the number of boxes between the two marks you have made.

TAKE HOME POINTS
Do not use an engineer's caliper with a wheel in the center. It will make it more difficult to adjust the caliper to the interval being measured.

Redrawn from Sole, Hartshorn, Lamborn: *Introduction to critical care nursing, ed 3*, Philadelphia, 2001, Saunders, p. 52.

Do You UNDERSTAND?

DIRECTIONS: **Fill in the blanks with the correct number of seconds.**

1. Each small box on the horizontal line equals _____ seconds.
2. Three small boxes on the horizontal line equals _____ seconds.
3. One large box on the horizontal line equals _____ seconds.
4. How long does it take for the QRS complex shown in the following figure to occur?

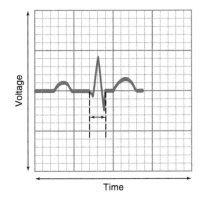

Answers: 1. 0.04; 2. 0.12; 3. 0.20; 4. 0.04 seconds × 2 = 0.08 seconds.

DIRECTIONS: **Fill in the correct word or number.**

5. Fifteen large boxes equal _____ seconds in time.

6. Second markers are located on the _____ or _____ margins of ECG paper.

7. Second markers can occur every 1, 3, or _____ seconds on ECG paper.

8. Five small boxes vertically from the baseline on the ECG paper equal _____ mm.

9. Decreased strength of heart contraction will result in decreased _____ of the ECG waveforms.

DIRECTIONS: **Look at the rhythm strip below and measure the points from A to E as indicated. Write your findings.**

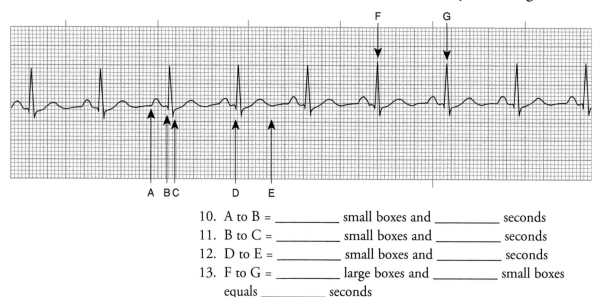

10. A to B = _____ small boxes and _____ seconds

11. B to C = _____ small boxes and _____ seconds

12. D to E = _____ small boxes and _____ seconds

13. F to G = _____ large boxes and _____ small boxes equals _____ seconds

What IS Documentation?

Documentation is usually performed by the health care provider at the beginning of each shift. In addition to documenting the various waveforms and intervals, you may be responsible for documenting the consistent, sustained rhythm of the patient's heart. You will gather this information by examining the patient's rhythm strip.

What You NEED TO KNOW

Most monitoring systems are computerized and include the patient's name, room number, date, time, heart rate, and lead in which the patient is being monitored. If this information is not recorded on the patient's rhythm strip, you need to write it in an area of the strip that is free of electrical tracing. You also need to verify that you ran and analyzed the strip by signing your name on the strip or in the patient's chart.

What You DO

When there is a change in the heart rhythm **(dysrhythmia),** you are responsible for printing a 6-second strip that includes the abnormality. You may also need to notify a physician (depending on the severity of the change). You should then document an entry in the patient's chart that includes the following:
- Date and time
- Rhythm change and analysis
- Patient assessment changes
- Treatment initiated
- Patient response to treatment
- Name of the health care provider who verified the rhythm

Do You UNDERSTAND?

Case Study

A 65-year-old man is admitted to your telemetry unit for acute exacerbation of asthma. His baseline vital signs are temperature 99° F, heart rate 110 beats/min, respiratory rate 22 breaths/min, and blood pressure (BP) 130/80 mm Hg. He has been in a sinus rhythm, but the alarms have just rung. When you enter the room, he is out of bed, sitting in a chair, and receiving his handheld nebulizer treatment of albuterol (Proventil). The monitor indicates that he has gone into a sinus tachycardia, with frequent, premature ventricular contractions.

He is complaining of palpitations and a flushed feeling. Vital signs are 100.4° F, 140, 36, BP 160/90 mm Hg. He is sweating and has an ashen color.

DIRECTIONS: **Give a sample of what you would document on the chart.**

_____

_____

_____

_____

_____

References

Boyer MJ: *Lippincott's need-to-know ECG facts,* Philadelphia, 1997, Lippincott.

Cummings RO: *ACLS provider manual,* Dallas, 2002, American Heart Association.

Dubin D: *Rapid interpretation of EKGs,* ed 6, Tampa, 2000, Cover Publishing.

Ehrat KS: *The art of EKG interpretation: a self-instructional text,* ed 4, Dubuque, IA, 1997, Kendall/Hunt.

Lewis KM: *Sensible ECG analysis,* Albany, NY, 2000, Delmar Publishing.

McHale JD, Carlson KK: *AACN procedure manual for critical care,* ed 4, Philadelphia, 2001, Saunders.

Paul S, Hebra JD: *The nurse's guide to cardiac rhythm interpretation: implications for patient care,* Philadelphia, 1997, Saunders.

Answer: **Date: 02/00; time: 1000. Calls patient's room. Finishes nebulizer of Proventil. Patient reports palpitation and flushed feeling, "I can't catch my breath." Patient is flushed, looks ashen, and is diaphoretic and warm to the touch. Vital signs: 100.4° F, 140, 36. Pulse is weak and thready. BP is elevated from normal by 30 mm Hg at 160/90 mm Hg. Pulse and respirations are elevated. Rhythm strip has changed from sinus rhythm to sinus tachycardia with premature ventricular contractions. Nebulizer treatment discontinued and patient assisted back to bed. Physician and nurse practitioner notified for further direction.**

NCLEX® Review

1. You are preparing a presentation on the basics of analyzing ECGs for a group of graduate nurses. Which of the following areas is most important to cover in your discussion?
   1 Voltage measurements
   2 Time measurements
   3 Use of calipers
   4 Heart size

2. A student nurse has measured Mr. O'Brien's QRS complex to be four small boxes wide. What time interval would this indicate?
   1 0.04 seconds
   2 0.20 seconds
   3 0.16 seconds
   4 1.4 seconds

3. While discussing changes on Ms. Laticia's ECG, you identify a waveform that measures five small boxes vertically on the ECG paper. This indicates:
   1 1 mm
   2 0.12 mm
   3 5 mm
   4 10 mm

4. Documentation on a rhythm strip should include all of the following except:
   1 Date and time
   2 Full name and title
   3 Signature of the reviewing physician
   4 Rhythm analysis

5. While reviewing Mr. Jackson's ECG, you find that his waveforms have increased in height. This may be an indication of which of the following conditions?
   1 Cardiac hypertrophy
   2 Cardiac tamponade
   3 Cardiac standstill
   4 Rheumatoid arthritis of the neck

NCLEX® Review Answers

1. 2 It is most important for the nurse to be able to accurately determine heart rate and regularity, which are time measurements. The other areas (voltage measurement, use of calipers, and heart size) are necessary to the discussion, but time measurements are the priority.

2. 3 0.16 seconds. Seven small boxes × 0.04 seconds (time allotted for each box) = 0.16 seconds.

3. 3 One small vertical block equals 1 mm. Therefore 1 mm times five small vertical blocks equals 5 mm.

4. 3 The physician or advanced practice nurse need not sign that he or she has reviewed the rhythm. Date, time, full name, title, and rhythm analysis are written either on the strip or in the health care provider's notes (or wherever hospital protocol dictates).

5. 1 Enlarged heart muscle (cardiac hypertrophy) causes an increase in numbers of vertical boxes and voltage on the ECG. Cardiac tamponade would decrease voltage, and cardiac standstill has no voltage. Rheumatoid arthritis would not affect the ECG.

Notes

Principles of Rhythm Interpretation Waveform Analysis

What You WILL LEARN

After reading this chapter, you will know how to do the following:
  ✔ Define depolarization.
  ✔ Identify normal waveforms.

To interpret a rhythm strip accurately, you must be able to identify waveforms correctly. In this chapter, waveform identification and the electrical events of depolarization and repolarization are discussed. The relationship of waveforms and intervals to the cardiac cycle are also covered.

What IS Depolarization?

Depolarization is an electrical event that can be recorded on the electrocardiographic (ECG) or rhythm strip. It is a process in which the positive ions (mainly potassium) move from inside the cell to an area of less concentration outside the cell. This loss of positively charged ions causes the inside of the myocardial cell to become more negative. Once the cell becomes stimulated, the cell membrane allows sodium to rush from the extracellular space to the intracellular space. This process results in a sudden change in electrical charge within the cell that can be recorded on the ECG as indicated by the P wave and QRS complex.

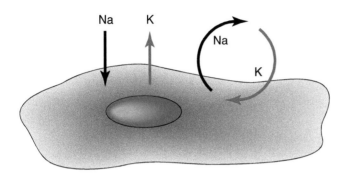

What You NEED TO KNOW

The movement of electrolytes stimulates cardiac cells. The ECG machine records the movement of sodium inside a cardiac cell at the same time that potassium moves out of the cell. Cardiac cells have the ability to conduct this current of energy from one cell to the next.

Electrodes placed on the chest and limbs pick up the electrical energy from this wave of depolarization. Depolarization normally begins in the sinoatrial (SA) node and moves through the atrium to the atrioventricular (AV) node, where there is a slight pause to allow both atria to contract. The wave then travels to the bundle of His, through the right and left bundle branches to the Purkinje fibers, and finally to the ventricular cells. The mechanical process of contraction usually follows the electrical process of depolarization within a few milliseconds (ms). (See Chapter 1 for a review of the conduction system.)

Rule of Electrical Flow

The waveforms on the ECG created by the process of depolarization may be positive, negative, or *isoelectric* (flat). One of the basic principles of electrocardiography explains the reason for positive, negative, or isoelectric waveforms. This principle states that if the energy from the depolarization process flows toward a positive recording electrode, the waveform will appear upright or positive.

Positive deflections

Negative deflections

Isoelectric line

Biphasic waveforms

If the energy from the depolarization process flows toward a negative recording electrode or away from a positive electrode, the waveform will appear as a negative deflection. If the energy is directed away from the positive and the negative electrode, there will be an isoelectric line recorded. A *biphasic waveform* (a two-phased waveform that goes up and down) occurs when the flow of energy is first directed toward a positive electrode and then toward a negative electrode (or vice versa).

What ARE the Waveforms in a Normal Cardiac Cycle?

On the ECG, one cardiac cycle is composed of a P wave, PR interval, QRS complex, ST segment, and T wave. These waveforms electrically represent one heart beat.

What You NEED TO KNOW

TAKE HOME POINTS
If conduction is normal, there should always be one P wave before every QRS complex.

P Wave

The *P wave* represents the firing of the SA node and atrial depolarization. It should be the first waveform in the cardiac cycle. Normally, P waves are upright, particularly in lead II. Both atria depolarize simultaneously, resulting in one P wave.

Normally, the P wave indicates that the SA node started the impulse that depolarized the atrium. If a P wave changes in shape, it may indicate that the impulse was initiated somewhere else in the atria or possibly in the junctional tissue, but outside the SA node.

In some abnormal rhythms, the atria may be stimulated more than once before the ventricles contract. In this case, there may be two or more P waves for each QRS complex.

In some abnormal rhythms or beats, the P wave may be completely absent.

Inverted P Wave

If a P wave is upside down (particularly in lead II where they are expected to be upright), it is considered inverted. *Inverted P waves* in lead II indicate that conduction through the atria occurred in an opposite, backward (**retrograde**) manner.

TAKE HOME POINTS

- A normal P wave is upright, rounded, and symmetric.
- There should be one P wave for every QRS complex.
- Whenever the P wave changes, note whether the change occurs with one beat or whether the entire rhythm has changed.

When this happens, the impulse originates in the AV junctional tissue, rather than in the SA node. In the normal heart, the SA node should always initiate the impulse and cause atrial depolarization, resulting in an upright P wave. Absent P waves, too many P waves, or inverted P waves compromise normal atrial contraction (atrial kick). The loss of synchronized, regular atrial contraction decreases the atrial contribution to ventricular filling and stretch, which reduces cardiac output.

PR Segment

The *PR segment* is an isoelectric (straight) line that occurs from the end of the P wave to the beginning of the QRS complex. The PR segment represents the delay of the electrical impulse at the AV node to allow atrial contraction.

PR Interval

The *PR interval* represents atrial depolarization and AV delay. It is measured from the beginning of the P wave to the end of the PR segment, which is the beginning of the QRS complex.

QRS Complex

The *QRS complex* represents ventricular depolarization. It may have a Q, R, or S wave, or it may have any combination of these waves.

Q Wave The *Q wave* is defined as the first negative deflection in the QRS complex. Not every QRS complex has a Q wave. Q waves may be considered a normal part of the QRS complex, or they may be considered to be significant, indicating that a myocardial infarction (MI) has occurred. The diagnosis of MI is based on many factors, including signs or symptoms, cardiac enzymes or markers, 12-lead ECG, and other tests (both invasive and noninvasive).

Q wave

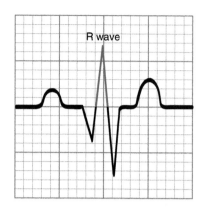

R Wave An *R wave* is the first positive deflection after the P wave. R waves may differ in size, ranging from tall to small to absent. QRS complexes may or may not have an R wave.

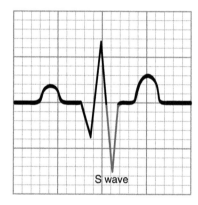

S Wave The *S wave* is also a negative wave. It is defined as the negative wave that follows the R wave or the second negative wave. As with other waves in the QRS complex, the S wave can be small, tall, or not there at all.

ST Segment

The *ST segment* is the line that follows the QRS complex and connects it to the T wave. It represents part of the ventricular repolarization process and, under normal circumstances, should be isoelectric.

T Wave

The *T wave* follows the QRS complex and represents ventricular repolarization. Changes in T wave amplitude can occur with electrolyte imbalances or ischemic processes to the myocardium. If you have difficulty finding P waves in heart rhythms that are very fast, look on top of the T wave.

There is a time during the resting state of the ventricle (during ventricular repolarization when the T wave occurs) when the cardiac cell is regaining a negative charge. This is called the *relative refractory period.*

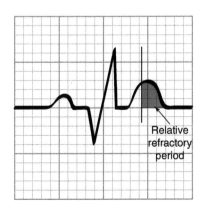

Any abnormal stimulus that occurs during the relative refractory period (e.g., an abnormal beat from the ventricles) could send the heart into electrical chaos.

U Wave

A *U wave* is a small waveform of unknown origin that may follow the T wave. If a U wave is present, it may have the same deflection as the T wave. U waves can be associated with electrolyte imbalances, particularly hypokalemia. (See *Saunders Nursing Survival Guide: Fluids & Electrolytes,* Chapter 5.)

QT Interval

The *QT interval* is measured from the beginning of the QRS complex to the end of the T wave. It represents the amount of time that it takes for ventricular depolarization and repolarization to occur. QT intervals vary with heart rate. Faster heart rates have shorter QT intervals, whereas slower heart rates have longer QT intervals.

Redrawn from Phipps, Sands, Marek: *Medical-surgical nursing: concepts and clinical practice,* ed 6, St Louis, 1999, Mosby, p. 675.

Certain antidysrhythmic drugs that prolong ventricular repolarization result in lengthened QT intervals. A life-threatening dysrhythmia can occur in patients with a lengthened QT interval. Treatment for this unique, polymorphic type of ventricular tachycardia, known as *torsade de pointes,* is aimed at shortening the refractory period (thus the QT interval) by interventions such as artificial overdrive pacing or the administration of intravenous (IV) isoproterenol, phenytoin, or lidocaine. Administration of magnesium has also shown beneficial results in terminating torsade de pointes.

Prolonged QT intervals have been associated with the life-threatening dysrhythmia, known as torsade de pointes, a unique, polymorphic type of ventricular tachycardia.

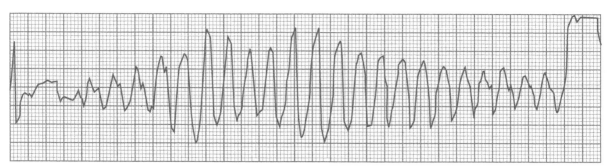

What You DO

- Assess your patient for any signs and symptoms (e.g., chest pain, shortness of breath, changes in consciousness level, changes in blood pressure) when a rhythm change occurs.
- Record a rhythm strip, and place it in the patient's chart for documentation.
- Note any antidysrhythmic medication the patient may be taking, and notify the prescribing professional.
- Follow accepted institution or advanced cardiac life support (ACLS) protocols for emergency interventions in patients with life-threatening dysrhythmias.

Do You UNDERSTAND?

DIRECTIONS: **What wave would each type of deflection produce?**

1. __B__ Positive
2. __C__ Negative
3. __D__ Biphasic
4. __A__ Isoelectric

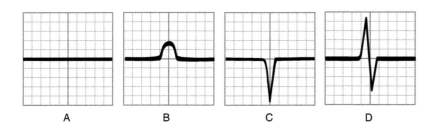

   A   B   C   D

DIRECTIONS: **Write the normal and abnormal characteristics of a P wave.**

5. Normal: _____

_____

_____

Answers: 1. B; 2. C; 3. D; 4. A; 5. Only one, upright, rounded, symmetric.

6. Abnormal: _____

_____

_____

DIRECTIONS: **Describe the normal Q, R, and S waves. What does the QRS complex indicate?**

7. Q wave: _____

8. R wave: _____

9. S wave: _____

10. QRS complex: _____

DIRECTIONS: **Label the electrocardiographic waves, intervals, and segments:**

11.

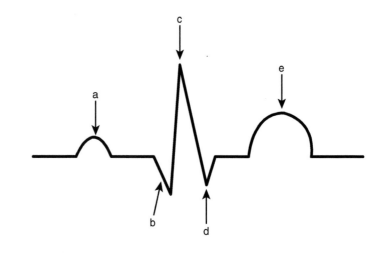

a. _____ b. _____ c. _____ d. _____ e. _____

12.

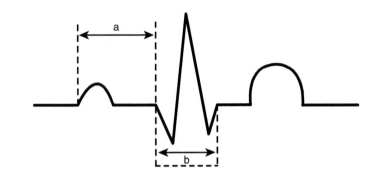

a. _____   b. _____

13.

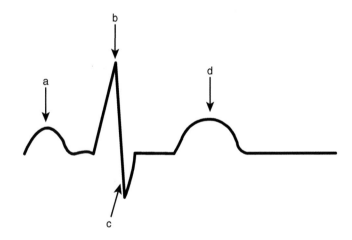

a. <u>P wave</u> b. <u>R wave</u> c. <u>S wave</u> d. <u>T wave</u>

14.

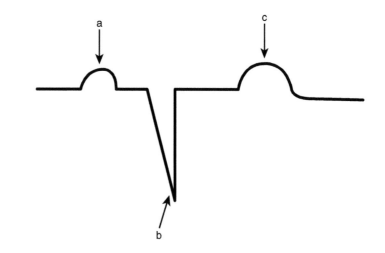

a. _____ b. _____ c. _____

15.

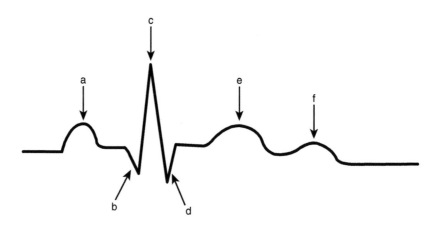

a. _____ b. _____ c. _____
d. _____ e. _____ f. _____

16.

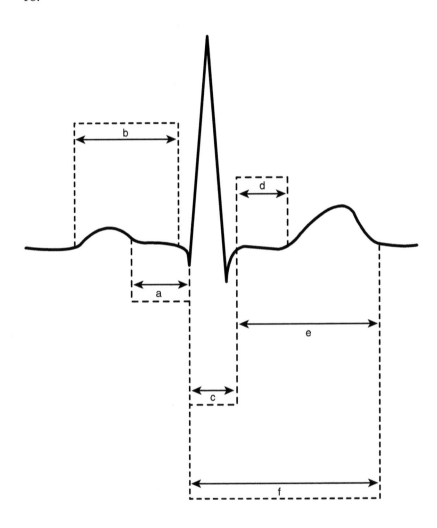

a. _____ b. _____ c. _____

d. _____ e. _____ f. _____

Remember that every QRS complex may or may not have a Q, R, and S wave.

Label the waveforms of the following QRS complexes:

17.

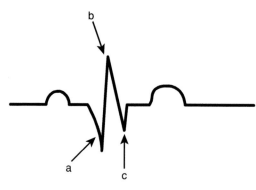

a. _____   b. _____   c. _____

18.

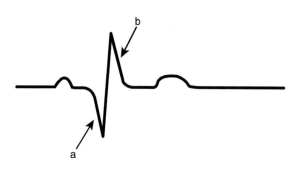

a. _____   b. _____

19.

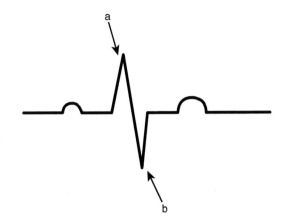

a. _____   b. _____

20.

_____

21.

_____

References

Aehlert B: *ECGs made easy,* ed 2, St Louis, 2002, Mosby.

American Heart Association: *Advanced cardiac life support provider manual,* Dallas, 1997, American Heart Association.

Boyer MJ: *Lippincott's need-to-know ECG facts,* Philadelphia, 1997, Lippincott.

Casey P: Management of patients with dysrhythmias and conduction problems. In Smeltzer S, Bare B, editors: *Bunner and Suddarth's textbook of medical-surgical nursing,* ed 9, Philadelphia, 2000, Lippincott.

Ehrat KS: *The art of EKG interpretation: a self-instructional text,* ed 4, Dubuque, IA, 1997, Kendall/Hunt.

Hartshorn JC, Sole ML, Lamborn ML: *Introduction to critical care nursing,* ed 3, Philadelphia, 2001, Saunders.

Huff J: *ECG workout: exercises in arrhythmia interpretation,* ed 3, Philadelphia, 1997, Lippincott.

Ignatavicius DD et al: *Medical-surgical nursing,* ed 3, Philadelphia, 1999, Saunders.

Lewis KM: *Sensible ECG analysis,* Albany, NY, 2000, Delmar Publishing.

Miracle VA, Sims JM: Making sense of the 12 lead ECG, *Nursing* 99(7):35, 1999.

Paul S, Hebra J: *The nurse's guide to cardiac rhythm interpretation: implications for patient care,* Philadelphia, 1998, Saunders.

Woods S: Dysrhythmia interpretation. In Sole LS, Lamborn ML, Hartshorn JC, editors: *Introduction to critical care nursing,* ed 3, Philadelphia, 2001, Saunders.

NCLEX® Review

1. The part of the rhythm that indicates the time it takes for the SA node to fire and the atria to depolarize is known as the:
   1 P wave
   2 R wave
   3 S wave
   4 T wave

2. The student you are tutoring is studying a rhythm strip. You know there is understanding when the student states:
   1 "There should be an isoelectric line after the PR interval."
   2 "P waves should be upright in lead II."
   3 "Q waves are always present in a QRS complex."
   4 "T waves are notched at their peak."

3. When the flow of electrical energy moves toward the positive electrode and then turns toward the negative, what waveform is recorded?
   1 Positive
   2 Negative
   3 Biphasic
   4 Isoelectric

4. The relative refractory period of the heart is:
   1 During the P wave
   2 In the middle of the R wave
   3 The first part of the S wave
   4 In the middle of the T wave

NCLEX® Review Answers

1. **1** P waves indicate atrial depolarization. R and S waves indicate ventricular depolarization. T waves indicate ventricular repolarization.

2. **2** P waves are positive in lead II because the positive electrode in lead II is below the heart and sees the normal atrial depolarization waves coming toward it. The PR interval is an isoelectric line. The QRS complex is after the PR interval.

Q waves are not always present in the QRS complex. T waves are normally rounded. Notching may indicate a P wave sitting on top of a T wave.

3. **3** A biphasic or two-phased waveform is caused when the wave of stimulation goes toward the positive and then the negative electrode. A positive waveform is caused when the electrical current flows toward a positive electrode. A negative waveform is caused by the wave of depolarization flowing toward the negative electrode. An isoelectric waveform is caused when the electrical flow is perpendicular or between a positive and negative electrode.

4. **4** The relative refractory period is the middle of the T wave. The T wave is ventricular repolarization and the middle of the T wave is where the cardiac cells try to regain their negativity. If stimulated here, the heart can go into electrical chaos. The P wave indicates atrial depolarization. The R and S waves indicate ventricular depolarization.

Notes

Chapter 4

Measuring Atrial and Ventricular Rates

What You WILL LEARN

After reading this chapter, you will know how to do the following:
- ✔ Describe the 6-Second Method.
- ✔ State the rule of 1500s.
- ✔ Differentiate between the rule of 300s and the rule of 1500s.

Now that you understand waveforms and how to measure time on electrocardiogram (ECG) paper, it is time to learn how to count atrial and ventricular rates on an ECG printout. In this chapter, three simple and rapid methods of estimating heart rate are described: (1) the 6-second method, (2) the rule of 1500s, and (3) the rule of 300s.

What IS the 6-Second Method?

The easiest method for counting atrial and ventricular rates is the 6-second method. This is also called the *rule of 10s.* The 6-second method is used for quick assessments when an approximate rate is needed, whether the heart rate is regular or irregular.

What You NEED TO KNOW

To determine heart rates using the 6-second method:
- Print out ECG paper covering a 6-second block of time (6-second strip).
- Remember to check the second markers on the top or bottom of the strip to identify a period of exactly 6 seconds. After every fifth large box is a 1-second marker, after every 15th large box there is a 3-second marker, and 6-second markers are after every 30th large box.

What You DO

To determine the **atrial rate** using the 6-second method:
- Count the number of P waves on a 6-second strip.
- Multiply that number by 10 to determine the full-minute rate. There are 10 6-second intervals in a minute.

To determine the **ventricular rate** using the 6-second method:

Count the number of R waves in a 6-second strip, and multiply that number by 10. The entire QRS complex must fit within the 6-second marks to count the R wave as a beat.

Example

In the following strip, the atrial rate is 60 beats per minute (bpm), because there are six P waves in the 6-second strip ($6 \times 10 = 60$). The ventricular rate is 60 bpm, because there are six QRS complexes in the 6-second strip ($6 \times 10 = 60$).

TAKE HOME POINTS
- Markers at the top or bottom of the strip will tell you over how many seconds an event has taken place.
- To identify a 6-second strip, it is important to check your ECG paper to see if markers occur every 1, 3, or 6 seconds. (See Chapter 2 for a review of second markers.)

The 6-second method will provide an estimate of your patient's heart rate. In a patient with a normal heart, the atrial and ventricular rates should be the same. This method can be used for patients with regular or irregular rhythms.

TAKE HOME POINTS
- A heart rate of above 100 is considered a tachycardia, and a heart rate below 60 is considered a bradycardia.
- When determining heart rate, the ventricular rate is preferred.
- The 6-second method is also referred to as the rule of 10s.

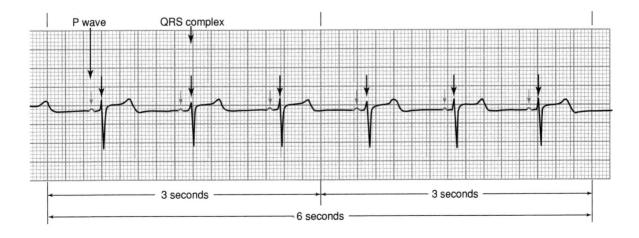

P wave   QRS complex

3 seconds   3 seconds

6 seconds

Do You UNDERSTAND?

DIRECTIONS: Use the 6-second rule to calculate the atrial and ventricular rates in strip 1 and strip 2.

1.

2.

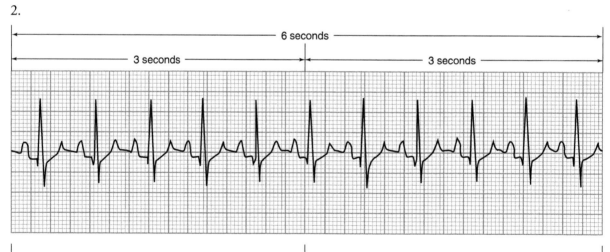

What IS the Rule of 1500s?

The *rule of 1500s* is a more accurate but slightly more complicated method for counting heart rates.

If the rhythm is a tachycardia or bradycardia, the patient needs to be assessed right away. Rates that are too slow or too fast can result in heart failure.

Answers: 1. Atrial rate is 70, because there are seven P waves in the 6-second strip; the ventricular rate is 70, because there are 7 complete QRS complexes in the 6-second strip; this is a normal rate; 2. There are 11 P waves in this 6-second strip; therefore the atrial rate is 110 (11 × 10 = 110); the ventricular rate is 110, because there are 11 QRS complexes in the 6-second strip; this is a tachycardia.

What You NEED TO KNOW

- The rule of 1500s may only be used for counting regular rhythms. A rhythm is considered regular when both the P waves and the QRS complexes are equally spaced.
- Atrial and ventricular rates should be equal in the normal heart.

What You DO

Atrial Rate

To determine the atrial rate using the rule of 1500s:
- Count the number of small blocks between the tallest point of two consecutive P waves.
- Divide that number (denominator) into 1500 (numerator).

Ventricular Rate

To determine the ventricular rate using the rule of 1500s:
- Count the number of small blocks between the peaks of two consecutive R waves.
- Divide this number into 1500.

Examine the following ECG strip. You will see that there are 23 small boxes between the last two P waves on the strip. If you want to determine the atrial rate using the rule of 1500s, you would divide 1500 by 23 (1500 ÷ 23 = 65). Therefore this strip indicates that the patient's atrial rate is 65 bpm.

> ! The rule of 1500s is used for determining rates only when the rhythm is regular. Atrial and ventricular rates should be equal in the normal heart.

3 seconds — 3 seconds — 6 seconds

TAKE HOME POINTS

Regardless of the method used to determine a patient's heart rate, always use the ventricular rate to analyze whether the rate is normal, fast, or slow.

To determine the ventricular rate using the rule of 1500s, count the small boxes between each R wave. In this case, there are 23 small boxes between each R wave on the strip. Once again, divide 1500 by 23. This means the ventricular rate indicated on the strip is also 65 bpm.

Do You UNDERSTAND?

DIRECTIONS: **Examine the next two rhythm-strip examples, and calculate the ventricular rates using the rule of 1500s.**

1.

2.

Answers: 1. **There are 25 small boxes between the R waves in this strip; therefore 1500 ÷ 25 = 60, or 60 bpm; this is a normal rate;** 2. **In this strip, there are 15 small boxes between the R waves; therefore 1500 ÷ 15 = 100, or 100 bpm; this is a normal rate.**

What IS the Rule of 300s?

The *rule of 300s* is a common method used to calculate regular heart rhythms. This method depends on observation and memorization. It is quick, simple, and does not require a calculator.

What You NEED TO KNOW

To use the rule of 300s, two sets of numbers must be memorized.

First set is 300, 150, and 100
Second set is 75, 60, and 50

Determine rate by observation

The heart rate can be determined by attaching these numbers to the heavy vertical lines between the peaks of two R waves. The theory behind the rule of 300s is that the distance between two heavy vertical lines is 1/300 of a minute. Therefore the number of large boxes between two R waves is divided into 300 to discover the rate per minute.

If the space between two R waves is three large boxes, 300 is divided by 3 (300 ÷ 3 = 100). This means that your patient's heart rate is 100 bpm. If the space between two R waves is eight large boxes, 300 is divided by 8 (300 ÷ 8 = 37). This means that your patient's heart rate is 37 bpm. You are not expected to memorize the numbers on the fine, vertical lines of the ECG; however, you should understand how to read them and use them to calculate your patient's heart rates. An additional set of numbers (43, 37, 33) can be used for slower rates. The 6-second method is easier to use when estimating slow heart rates (rates below 50 bpm).

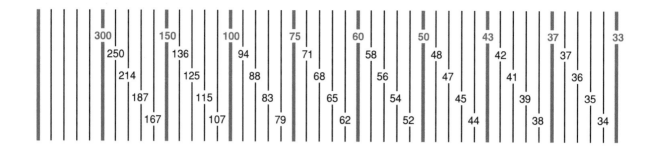

What You DO

- Find an R wave that peaks on a heavy vertical line.
- Name that line "Start."
- Name each consecutive heavy vertical line according to the numbers that you have memorized until you have reached the second R wave. See the following examples:

1.

TAKE HOME POINTS

- The rule of 300s provides an estimation of heart rate, not the exact heart rate.
- If the second R wave does not fall exactly on the heavy line, use the number on the heavy line closest to it.

The rule of 300s should only be used to calculate the heart rates of those with regular heart rhythms.

Heart rate ≈ 60

2.

Heart rate ≃ 37

3.

Heart rate is less than 100 and slightly greater than 75 (it is ≃ 80).

TAKE HOME POINTS

- Remember, "Start"; then 300, 150, 100; then 75, 60, 50.
- If your patient's heart rate is below 50, it is easier to go to the 6-second method.
- It is not necessary to memorize the numbers on the fine vertical lines of the ECG strip.

www.americanheart.org

www.atlcard.com

www.wices.com/

icescardiac

Do You UNDERSTAND?

DIRECTIONS: **Estimate the heart rate on the following rhythm strip using the rule of 300s.**

1.

References

Cummings RO: *ACLS provider manual,* Dallas, 2002, American Heart Association.

Dubin D: *Rapid interpretation of EKGs,* ed 5, Tampa, 1996, Cover Publishing.

Ignatavicius DD et al: *Medical-surgical nursing,* ed 3, Philadelphia, 1999, Saunders.

Johns C: Arrhythmias. In Lewis SM, Heitkemper HH, Dirksen SR: *Medical-surgical nursing,* ed 5, St Louis, 2000, Mosby.

Paul S, Hebra J: *The nurse's guide to cardiac rhythm interpretation: implications for patient care,* Philadelphia, 1998, Saunders.

Scrima D: Foundations of arrhythmia interpretation, *Medsurg Nurs* 6:4, 1997.

Woods S: Dysrhythmia interpretation. In Sole LS, Lamborn ML, Hartshorn JC, editors: *Introduction to critical care nursing,* ed 3, Philadelphia, 2001, Saunders.

Answer: **1. Heart rate is approximately 80.**

NCLEX® Review

1. When determining heart rate in a normal heart, you should remember that the atrial rate is:
   1. Always slower than the ventricular rate
   2. The preferred rate to measure
   3. Always faster than the ventricular rate
   4. Always equal to the ventricular rate

2. When discussing the estimated methods of heart-rate calculation with a group of students, which of the following methods would you identify as most accurate?
   1. Six-second method
   2. Rule of 1500s
   3. Rule of 300s
   4. Rule of 5s

3. The 6-second method is the only method of rate calculation that can be used for:
   1. Measuring regular and irregular heart rates
   2. Measuring R-to-R time intervals
   3. Measuring P-to-P time intervals
   4. Measuring small boxes

4. Mr. Sylvester's heart rate is 120 beats per minute. You would be correct in describing this rate as a:
   1. Bradycardia
   2. Normal rate
   3. Tachycardia
   4. Heart block

5. Using the 6-second method or the rule of 10s, which of the following is the atrial rate if the number of P waves on a 6-second strip is 5?
   1. 300
   2. 30
   3. 50
   4. 25

NCLEX® Review Answers

1. 4 In the normal heart, the atrial and ventricular rates should be equal. An atrial rate slower than the ventricular rate would indicate bradycardia. Ventricular rates, not atrial rates, are the preferred rate to measure because they are more easily identified. An atrial rate faster than the ventricular rate would indicate tachycardia.

2. 2 The rule of 1500s gives a precise heart rate. The 6-second method is for a quick estimation of rates and can be used for both regular and irregular rhythms. The rule of 300s can be performed without a calculator and is used to calculate approximate rates for regular rhythms only. There is no rule of 5s.

3. 1 The 6-second method looks at number of beats and therefore can be used to determine rates for regular and irregular rhythms. Measuring R-to-R intervals and P-to-P intervals and counting only small boxes can be done with the rule of 1500s or the rule of 300s.

4. 3 Rates greater than 100 are described as tachycardia. A bradycardia is a heart rate below 60. A normal rate is between 60 and 100. A heart block involves looking at the PR interval and its relationship to the QRS.

5. 3 10×5 (number of P waves) = 50.

Notes

5

Analyzing the Rhythm Strip

What You WILL LEARN

After reading this chapter, you will know how to do the following:

- ✔ Describe the 8-Step Method.
- ✔ Describe what knowledge you need to determine rhythm regularity.
- ✔ Describe a PR Interval Measurement.
- ✔ Explain the knowledge you need to fully assess a QRS Complex.
- ✔ State what measurement of the QT interval represents.
- ✔ List one patient condition associated with an ST segment change and another one with a T wave change.
- ✔ Describe two signs or symptoms that may be associated with a dysrhythmia.

The previous chapters have discussed waveforms, electrocardiographic (ECG) paper, and measuring atrial and ventricular rates. Now you are ready to apply this information to analyzing a rhythm strip. This chapter covers a step-by-step approach to rhythm strip interpretation, known as the 8-step method.

What IS the 8-Step Method?

The *8-step method* of interpreting rhythms is a good way to identify the origin of an impulse on a rhythm strip, describe the conduction sequence of the rhythm, and define the salient features of the rhythm. To interpret information on a rhythm strip using this method, you would take the following eight steps:

1. Identify the waveforms and assess the morphology and location of the P waves, QRS complexes, and T waves.
2. Count the atrial rate. — P wave
3. Count the ventricular rate. R wave
4. Determine whether the atrial rhythm is regular or irregular.
5. Determine whether the ventricular rhythm is regular or irregular.
6. Measure the PR interval to determine whether it is within normal limits, and ensure that all of the PR intervals are consistent.
7. Measure the width of the QRS complex to determine whether it is within normal limits. Ensure that all the QRS complexes are consistent.
8. Assess the clinical significance of the rhythm.

What You NEED TO KNOW

To complete the first step of rhythm strip analysis (identification of the waveforms), you should ask the following questions:

- Is there one P wave before every QRS complex?
- Is the P wave upright in lead II?
- Do all the P waves look alike or have the same shape?
- Can the waveforms representing ventricular depolarization be identified (the QRS complex)?
- Is there a Q, R, or an S wave present?
- Do all the QRS complexes look alike?
- Can the T waves be identified? Do all the T waves look alike?

Once you have identified the waveforms, you should count the atrial and ventricular rates (see Chapter 4). Next, you should determine whether the atrial rhythm is regular. To do this, you should measure P-to-P intervals. A regular atrial rhythm is one in which each P-to-P interval plots out the same distance.

TAKE HOME POINTS

- The 8-step method looks at rate, rhythm, conduction times, and the clinical significance of the rhythm.
- It is essential to compare all intervals in the rhythm to each other to make sure they are consistent.
- P waves should occur before the QRS complex.
- T waves should follow the QRS complex.
- In most cases, the QRS complex is the largest waveform in the rhythm strip. (Therefore you should look for P waves where they are supposed to be: in front of the QRS complex.)
- Remember, if the rhythm is fast, P waves may be sitting on top of the T waves.
- Because the sinoatrial (SA) node should initiate the impulse and conduct to the ventricles, there should be one P wave before every QRS complex. Therefore the atrial and ventricular rates should be the same.

What You DO

Atrial regularity is determined by plotting P-to-P intervals using calipers.

- Place the left caliper tip at the beginning of the P wave, and place the right caliper tip at the beginning of the very next P wave. This is the P-to-P interval.
- Without changing the width of the caliper tips, lift the calipers and place them on the next P wave.
- If the caliper tips fall on the next P wave, the atrial rhythm is considered regular.
- If the caliper tips do not fall on the next P wave (off more than one small block), the atrial rhythm is considered irregular.

Do You UNDERSTAND?

DIRECTIONS: **Measure the P-to-P intervals in the examples that follow. Is the atrial rhythm regular or irregular?**

1.

Answers: 1. **Regular; therefore the atrial rhythm is regular.**

2.

What IS Determining the Ventricular Rhythm?

The next step is to determine whether the ventricular rhythm is regular or irregular. A regular ventricular rhythm reveals whether the ventricles are firing in a normal, even manner.

What You NEED TO KNOW

Determining the regularity of the ventricular rhythm is similar to determining atrial rhythm. However, instead of measuring P-to-P intervals, the R-to-R intervals are measured (QRS complex to QRS complex).

What You DO

Measuring ventricular regularity (rhythm) is similar to measuring atrial rhythm. However, the R-to-R intervals are measured, instead of the P-to-P intervals.

- Use calipers.
- Place the right caliper tip on top of an R wave and the left tip on top of the next R wave.
- Without changing the width of the caliper tips, lift the calipers and place them on the next R wave.
- If the caliper tips fall on the next R wave, the ventricular rhythm is considered regular.
- If the caliper tips do not fall on the next R wave (off more than one small block), the ventricular rhythm is considered irregular.

Do You UNDERSTAND?

DIRECTIONS: **Measure the R-to-R intervals in the following examples. Is the ventricular rhythm regular or irregular?**

1.

2.

What IS PR Interval Measurement

Once you have determined the ventricular rhythm, it is time to determine whether the PR interval measurement is within normal limits. The PR interval includes the time it takes for atrial depolarization and AV holding to occur.

What You NEED TO KNOW

A normal PR interval is between 0.12 and 0.20 seconds (between three and five small boxes on the ECG paper).

TAKE HOME POINTS

If the PR interval is less than 0.12 seconds or greater than 0.20 seconds, it is abnormal.

What You DO

You should measure the PR interval from the beginning of the P wave to the end of the PR segment, which is the beginning of the QRS complex.

Do You UNDERSTAND?

DIRECTIONS: **Identify the PR intervals in the following examples, and identify the abnormal PR intervals.**

1.

2.

3.

4.

What IS Assessing the QRS Complex?

The QRS complex represents ventricular depolarization. After determining whether the PR interval is normal, the QRS complex is assessed to see whether it is within normal limits.

What You NEED TO KNOW

The QRS complex may have a Q, an R, or an S wave (or any combination of these waves).

TAKE HOME POINTS

A QRS complex of 0.12 seconds wide or wider indicates that the rhythm originates in the ventricles or that some interventricular conduction delay has occurred.

Answers: 3, 0.14 seconds; 4, 0.24 seconds (abnormal).

What You DO

- You should measure a QRS complex from the end of the PR interval, which is the waveform that begins the QRS complex and includes all of the waveforms that represent ventricular depolarization.
- A normal QRS complex should be less than 0.12 seconds or fewer than three small boxes on the ECG paper.

Do You UNDERSTAND?

DIRECTIONS: **Measure the duration of the QRS complex in the following examples, and identify the abnormal QRS complexes.**

1.

2.

3.

4.

What IS Measurement
of the QT Interval?

The QT interval represents the amount of time that it takes for ventricular depolarization and repolarization to occur. Although measurement of the QT interval is not always included in the 8-step method of rhythm interpretation, it is important to note a baseline QT interval.

What You NEED TO KNOW

Normal QT intervals are rate dependent, and most measure between 0.36 and 0.44 seconds. (See the following examples of QT interval measurement.)

1. QT interval = 0.34 seconds (abnormal)

2. QT interval = 0.34 seconds (abnormal)

3. QT interval = 0.44 seconds (abnormal)

4. QT interval = 0.36 seconds (abnormal)

What IS the Significance of the ST Segment and T Wave?

Normally, the ST segment is an isoelectric line that begins at the end of the QRS complex and ends at the beginning of the T wave.

What You NEED TO KNOW

ST segment depression occurs when the ST segment is deflected downward. If the ST segment is deflected upward, it is referred to as ST segment elevation. ST segment elevation or depression can be significant if the change is more than one small box (1 millimeter) upward or downward in two or more leads that look at one surface area of the heart. Based on the patient's clinical presentation and lab values ST segment elevation can indicate acute myocardial injury, pericarditis, variant (Prinzmetal) angina due to coronary artery spasm, or ventricular aneurysm. ST segment depression can indicate ischemia, digitalis effect, or reciprocal changes associated with an acute myocardial infarction.

T waves usually are upright and normal height. Tall, peaked T waves may be an indication of hyperkalemia. Often, if the QRS originates in the ventricles, the T wave will be deflected in the opposite direction of the QRS complex. Also, inverted T waves may indicate myocardial ischemia.

TAKE HOME POINTS

When trying to evaluate changes on the electrocardiogram, always consider the patient's clinical presentation, signs/symptoms, such as chest pressure, pain, and/or shortness of breath. Lab values and other diagnostic tools should also be considered.

What IS the Significance of the Rhythm?

The final step in rhythm-strip analysis is to determine the clinical significance of the rhythm. This is an essential step in evaluating the patient's condition.

What You DO

Notify the health care professional if your patient experiences any signs or symptoms of instability. You should be prepared to treat the rhythm, based on your institution's protocols.

If a patient experiences any signs or symptoms of instability, such as hypotension, light-headedness, shortness of breath, chest pain, or changes in levels of consciousness, you should notify the health care professional and be prepared to treat the rhythm, based on your institution's protocols.

Do You UNDERSTAND?

DIRECTIONS: **Examine the following rhythm strips. Using the 8-step method, note the following characteristics: location and shape of waveforms, atrial rate, ventricular rate, atrial and ventricular rhythms, PR interval, and QRS complex width. You should also practice measuring QT intervals.**

1.

2.

3.

4.

5.

DIRECTIONS: **Fill in the blanks.**

6. Using calipers to measure from P wave to P wave determines

   _____ _____.

7. Using calipers to measure from QRS (R wave) to QRS (R wave)
   determines _____ _____.

8. Measuring from the beginning of the P wave to the beginning of
   the QRS complex determines the _____ _____.

9. The measurement from the end of PR interval to the beginning of
   the ST segment is called the _____.

10. List three symptoms that may be associated with rhythm changes
    that are clinically significant.

References

Aehlert B: *ECGs made easy*, ed 2, St Louis, 2002, Mosby.

American Heart Association: *Advanced cardiac life support provider manual*, Dallas,
1997, American Heart Association.

Ignatavicius DD et al: *Medical-surgical nursing*, ed 3, Philadelphia, 1999, Saunders.

Paul S, Hebra J: *The nurse's guide to cardiac rhythm interpretation: implications for
patient care*, Philadelphia, 1998, Saunders.

Woods S: Dysrhythmia interpretation. In Sole LS, Lamborn ML, Hartshorn JC,
editors: *Introduction to critical care nursing*, ed 3, Philadelphia, 2001, Saunders.

Answers: 6. atrial regularity; 7. ventricular regularity; 8. PR interval; 9. QRS complex; 10. hypotension, chest pain, shortness of breath, changes in levels of consciousness, or light-headedness.

NCLEX® Review

1. When using the 8-step method, you should look at configuration and location of which of the following?
   1 P waves
   2 PR interval
   3 ST segments
   4 Absolute refractory period

2. Conduction times in ECG analysis refer to:
   1 P waves
   2 PR interval
   3 ST segments
   4 P-to-P interval

3. A health care provider you are tutoring shows you a rhythm strip that has been run on a new patient with unstable angina. To help analyze this strip, the best thing to tell the provider is:
   1 "Don't worry. Just put it on the chart, and call it to the physician's attention during rounds this morning."
   2 "Try to describe the rhythm using as much descriptive language as possible."
   3 "Give it to me, and I will do the analysis."
   4 "The ECG technician will help you with it in a minute."

NCLEX® Review Answers

1. 1 The configuration and location of P waves that look the same indicate the rhythm is coming from the SA node. P waves that are inverted or notched are usually from an ectopic focus. The PRI is a measure of conduction. The ST segment is not viewed solely from a rhythm strip; a 12-lead ECG must be examined. The absolute refractory period is located in the middle of the T wave; this is examined in relationship to an R wave.

2. 2 The PR interval is indicative of conduction above the ventricle conduction. The P waves are not measured in length alone. They are, however, part of the PRI, which is a measurement of conduction. The ST segments are not measured for time; they are measured up and down in a 12-lead ECG. The P-to-P interval is measured to determine atrial regularity.

3. 2 Even if the health care provider does not know exactly what the rhythm is, he or she needs to go through the steps to tell what characteristics the rhythm has so that he or she can more fully describe the rhythm to other health care practitioners. Telling a provider "not to worry" is belittling; rather, he or she should be given every opportunity to learn the correct way to determine rhythm strips. Doing it for the provider will not help the learning process. He or she needs to practice under direct supervision. The ECG technician, although a good resource person, is not the legal professional in charge of the patient's care.

Troubleshooting Problems in Waveforms

What You WILL LEARN

After reading this chapter, you will know how to do the following:

✔ Define artifact.
✔ Describe what artifact looks like.
✔ Define 60-cycle interference.
✔ Describe weak signal.

To analyze an electrocardiographic (ECG) recording accurately, it is necessary to have a clear, well-produced tracing with a stationary isoelectric baseline **(baseline without drift).** Common technical problems that require troubleshooting artifact include 60-cycle interference, weak signals, wandering baselines, chaotic tracings, and artificial interference. Other important troubleshooting issues include loss of signal, excessive artifacts, and falsely elevated heart rates. In this chapter, the recognition of artifact is discussed, and tips for troubleshooting waveform problems are provided.

What IS Artifact?

Artifact is an artificial disturbance of the ECG signal that interferes with high-quality capture of the ECG tracing.

Often, artifact is caused by electrical interference **(60-cycle interference),** muscular activity, movement, or mechanical problems.

Artifact can be compared with the noise you hear when making tuning adjustments to a radio. These signal distortions may be continual or intermittent.

What You NEED TO KNOW

One of the most common causes of artifact is patient movement. Hiccups, shivering, convulsions, and chest movements that occur during respirations can interfere with waveforms and cause the baseline of the ECG tracing to wander.

The following ECG strip demonstrates artifact resulting from patient movement. This type of interference may trigger the monitor's heart-rate alarm.

⚠ Patient movements cause interference that may trigger the monitor's heart-rate alarm.

What You DO

When an ECG artifact is discovered, you need to do the following:
- Assess the patient, and ensure his or her safety.
- Differentiate between a patient problem and a mechanical problem by working in an organized fashion, from the patient back to the monitoring system.
- If the patient is in any distress, initiate further assessment and treatment if necessary.
- Ensure that the electrode pads and lead wires are attached to the patient. Patient movement can cause electrodes and lead wires to detach. Keep in mind that they should be changed and repositioned every 3 days (sooner if problematic).

- Inspect the lead wires for corrosion or worn areas. Normally, lead wires are cleaned and reused between patients. However, if they are corroded or frayed, they should be discarded and replaced.
- Work with one piece of equipment at a time, checking for a clean tracing between each intervention. For persistent problems, a portable monitor may be needed to monitor the rhythm at the bedside while troubleshooting.

TAKE HOME POINTS

- The alarm system is a critical safety feature!
- Never turn off or ignore alarms!
- Always assess your patient first.

What IS 60-Cycle Interference?

Interference that is attributed to improper grounding of electrical equipment placed near the patient is known as *60-cycle* or *alternating current* (AC) *interference*. The result of this type of interference is a wide, fuzzy baseline.

TAKE HOME POINTS

If unable to find the source of the ECG artifact, call the appropriate biomedical or maintenance personnel and have them check the equipment for potential hazards or defects.

What You NEED TO KNOW

The hallmarks of this type of artifact are 60 small, regular spikes in a 1-second interval tracing.

What You DO

When you discover an ECG with 60-cycle interference, do the following:

- Assess the patient, and ensure his or her safety.

If the patient is on mechanical ventilation that has no battery back-up, ensure that oxygen delivery and ventilation are provided by Ambu bag before you assess the plug. Ensure that there is battery back-up when troubleshooting intravenous (IV) pump plugs. The delivery of IV vasoactive and antiarrhythmic drugs should not be interrupted during troubleshooting.

- Unplug one piece of electrical equipment at a time, and note whether the tracing clears when the equipment is unplugged.
- Once you have determined which piece of equipment is responsible for the interference, you should plug it into a different outlet.
- Check to see whether any new equipment has been added to the bedside, such as electric shavers or radios brought from home. This type of equipment should be evaluated by the biomedical department to determine whether it is responsible for the interference.
- If the equipment continues to cause interference when placed in the new location, replace it.
- Send any defective equipment to the biomedical department for inspection and repair.

TAKE HOME POINTS

Often, electrical interference is caused by a damaged plug on the patient's bed.

Do You UNDERSTAND?

DIRECTIONS: **On the lines provided, list four possible causes for artifacts.**

1. _____
   _____
   _____
   _____

DIRECTIONS: **On the lines provided, list the steps you would take to troubleshoot an artifact problem.**

2. _____
   _____
   _____
   _____
   _____
   _____
   _____

Answers: 1. Hiccups, shivering, convulsions, strong respiratory movements; 2. Assess the patient and ensure safety, initiate further assessment and treatment (if necessary), check to see that electrode pads and lead wires are attached to patient, inspect lead wires and clean or replace (if necessary), send any faulty equipment to the biomedical department.

What IS a Weak Signal?

Occasionally, the monitor will not pick up the patient's actual heart rate because of a *weak signal*. This may be caused by an improperly placed, loose, or dry electrode. Weak signals may also be caused by obesity, because electrical impulse from the patient's heart must travel through a greater amount of subcutaneous tissue to reach the electrode.

What You NEED TO KNOW

The QRS (the largest waveform) must be a certain height for the monitor to count it as a heartbeat. In some conditions, such as cardiac tamponade, the mechanical compression of the heart may prevent a strong heartbeat. However, keep in mind that the QRS complex may appear too small if the health care provider has forgotten to turn up the gain or the size-adjustment knob, which makes the complex height taller.

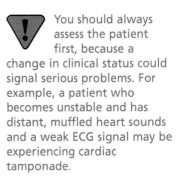

You should always assess the patient first, because a change in clinical status could signal serious problems. For example, a patient who becomes unstable and has distant, muffled heart sounds and a weak ECG signal may be experiencing cardiac tamponade.

What You DO

When you discover a weak signal, do the following:
- Assess the patient to determine whether there is any change in his or her condition.
- Systematically check the electrodes, connections, and lead wires for any damage.
- Count the patient's apical heart rate for 1 minute, and compare it with the rate on the monitor.
- Turn the gain or size-adjustment knob up until the monitor picks up each heartbeat.
- Change the lead select button on the monitoring system to a lead that allows better visualization of the heart rhythm.

TAKE HOME POINTS

To ensure proper functioning of the monitoring system, the patient's apical heart rate should be checked and compared against the rate reported on the monitor.

What ARE Other Types of Artifact?

Other types of artifact include a wandering baseline, chaotic tracings, and factitious (artificial) interference.

What You NEED TO KNOW

A *wandering baseline* can cause problems in the analysis of ECG recording. The baseline of the patient's rhythm is determined by drawing a flat line through the ECG complex.

When the patient is restless or breathing heavily, the baseline will not be straight. Rather, it will appear to ride up and down in a wavy manner.

⚠ The up and down movement of the baseline can make it difficult to obtain accurate measurements when assessing the rhythm strip, which can lead to misinterpretation.

Often a wandering baseline is caused by chest movement that occurs during respiration. Anxiety or pain may contribute to a wandering baseline.

Chaotic tracings have many spikes and dips, which interfere with the underlying complexes. This usually results from poor electrode contact from dried electrode gel, loose lead wires, or cable problems.

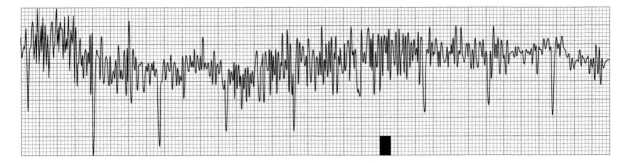

Factitious interference is produced by movement of the equipment or lead wires, such as a patient tapping or pulling on the wires or a patient brushing his teeth and causing movement of the telemetry monitor.

What You DO

- Remember to always assess the patient first. Patients should be assessed for unusual movement.
- If your patient is experiencing pain, you should evaluate the pain and institute appropriate pain-relieving measures, including medication and positioning.
- Document your assessment, interventions, and patient response.
- Ensure that the electrode gel is moist and intact.
- Ensure that lead wires and cables are operational and not fractured.
- Reposition any electrodes that have been placed over bony areas or areas of skin that move during respiration. If electrodes are placed on your patient's arms and legs, it may help to bring them closer to the heart.
- Continue to maintain the placement area required for the lead wire.
- Ensure appropriate patient education on the purpose of cardiac monitoring.

TAKE HOME POINTS

The lead wires and cables should not be so tight that they pull on the electrodes.

• If the artifact continues after patient assessment and equipment troubleshooting, contact the biomedical/technical support department in your institution.

Type of Artifact	Troubleshooting
60-cycle interference	Assess for the following: • Damaged lead wires • Poor electrode contact • Improper grounding • Current leakage from other electrical equipment
Weak signals	Assess for damaged lead wires or poor electrode contact. Change electrode position. Change lead selection.
Wandering baseline	Reposition any electrodes that have been placed over bony areas or areas of skin that move during respiration. If electrodes are placed on your patient's arms and legs, it may help to bring them closer to the heart.
Chaotic tracings	Assess for dried electrode gel, loose lead wires, or cable problems.
Artificial interference	Ensure patient education on purpose/intent of cardiac monitoring and what types of movement may cause artifacts.

OTHER TRACING ISSUES

Loss of signal due to electrode detachment	Always assess patient's clinical status first! Replace missing electrodes, lead wires.
Falsely elevated heart rates—monitor is sensing both the QRS complex and T wave for counting heart rate (double counting)	Reduce the gain (voltage). Reposition electrodes. Select a different lead for monitoring.
Excessive artifact with small amplitude signals	Assess for weak battery in telemetry monitor.

Do You UNDERSTAND?

DIRECTIONS: Define the following types of artifact.

1. Weak signal: _____

_____

_____

Answer: 1. A weak signal is an ECG complex that is not picked up when the monitor counts the patient's heart rate.

2. AC (60-cycle) interference:

_____

_____

3. Wandering baseline:

_____

_____

4. Artifact:

_____

_____

DIRECTIONS: **Unscramble the words in parentheses to fill in the blanks.**

5. To ensure proper functioning of the cardiac-monitoring system, you should always compare the heart rate on the ECG with the patient's _____ pulse. *(ipaacl)*

6. If a patient's ECG has a wandering baseline, the electrodes may have been placed over an area of _____. *(vmomeent)*

DIRECTIONS: **Identify the following types of artifact:**

7.

8.

9.

10.

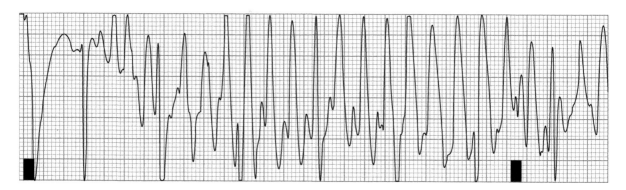

References

Aehlert B: *ECGs made easy*, ed 2, St Louis, 2002, Mosby.

American Heart Association: *Advanced cardiac life support provider manual*, Dallas, 1997, American Heart Association.

Bloomquist J, Love M: Cardiovascular assessment and diagnostic procedures. In Urden L, Stacy K, editors: *Priorities in critical care*, ed 3, St Louis, 2000, Mosby.

Huff J: *ECG workout: exercises in arrhythmia interpretation*, ed 3, Philadelphia, 1997, Lippincott.

Paul S, Hebra J: *The nurse's guide to cardiac rhythm interpretation: implications for patient care*, Philadelphia, 1998, Saunders.

Woods S: Dysrhythmia interpretation. In Sole LS, Lamborn ML, Hartshorn JC, editors: *Introduction to critical care nursing*, ed 3, Philadelphia, 2001, Saunders.

NCLEX® Review

1. When a patient's ECG alarm goes off because of a suggested artifact, your first action should be to:
   1 Ignore the warning.
   2 Call the prescribing professional in charge of the patient and ask for an interpretation of the rhythm strip.
   3 Assess the patient to ensure his or her safety.
   4 Ask a more experienced provider for direction.

2. A wandering baseline is caused by:
   1 Improperly grounded electrical equipment
   2 A monitor that does not count each QRS
   3 Chest movement during respiration
   4 Shivering from a high fever

3. Which of the following is not a cause of artifact?
   1 Hiccup
   2 Convulsions
   3 Shivering
   4 Tachycardia

4. A cause of 60-cycle interference is:
   1 Jumping up and down
   2 An ungrounded electrical shaver
   3 A straight razor
   4 A battery-operated radio

NCLEX® Review Answers

1. 3 A health care provider should always check the patient first if the monitor alarm sounds. Alarms should never be ignored. The physician or advanced practice nurse only needs to be called if the patient requires medical treatment for a change in rhythm. The advice of a more experienced provider is not needed until the situation is assessed and found to be beyond your ability to understand.

2. 3 Chest movements up and down during respiration will cause the rhythm strip to move up and down in a regular cyclic pattern. Improperly grounded electrical equipment causes 60-cycle interference (electrical). Weak signals may cause the monitor to miss QRS complexes and therefore record a falsely low heart rate. High fevers can cause artifact or the pick-up of muscular tremors.

3. 4 Tachycardia is a fast heart rate and not artifact. Hiccups, convulsions, and shivering can cause artifact because they cause strong muscular movements.

4. 2 An ungrounded electrical device (in this case, a shaver) can cause leakage of electrical current and therefore electrical interference. Jumping up and down will cause muscular interference. A straight razor and a battery-operated radio do not run on electrical current and therefore are acceptable for patient use.

Notes

Chapter

7

Electrocardiogram: Monitoring and Electrode Placement

What You WILL LEARN

After reading this chapter, you will know how to do the following:

- ✔ Describe what a chest lead is.
- ✔ Explain the primary purpose of a 12-lead ECG.
- ✔ Define continuous ECG monitoring.
- ✔ Define a 3-Lead System.
- ✔ Explain the difference between a chest lead and a modified chest lead (MCL).
- ✔ Differentiate a 5-lead system from a 3-lead system.
- ✔ Explain selection of a monitoring lead and its importance to patient care.

In this chapter, the differences between continuous bedside monitoring and 12-lead monitoring are discussed. You will also learn how to place electrodes on a patient.

The *electrocardiogram* (ECG) is a graphic display of the electrical activity of the heart. Electrical activity, depolarization, and repolarization can be picked up by electrodes placed on the skin. This electrical activity is transmitted via lead wires to a monitoring device. The monitoring device converts the electrical activity into a graphic waveform (oscilloscope) display. An oscilloscope is the part of the monitor that magnifies (over 1000 times) the electrical activity of the heart and displays it as a continuous waveform recording on the monitor screen.

What ARE the Components of the ECG Equipment?

Leads

The word *lead* can have two different meanings. First, it can refer to the small, flexible, color-coded wires leading from the electrodes to the monitoring device. These leads are coded with letters on the head of the wire, and the colors indicate where they are to be placed on the body:

Letters	Meaning	Color
RA	Right arm	White
LA	Left arm	Black
RL	Right leg	Green
LL	Left leg	Red

There may also be a C lead (which indicates "chest") on some systems. The C lead is always brown.

The word *lead* can also refer to the standardized patterns of electrode placement. Electrodes are placed on different parts of the body (chest, arms, legs) to allow the electrical activity of the heart to be viewed from different angles. These *leads* are discussed in detail later in this chapter.

www.americanheart.org
www.atlcard.com/
introekg.html
www.wices.com/
icescardiac

Electrodes

Electrodes are small, sticky discs or tabs that are strategically placed on the patient's chest and extremities. They pick up and transmit the *millivolts* (mV) of electrical energy produced by the heart during depolarization and repolarization via the lead wire to a monitoring device. Disc-shaped electrodes have an inner, moist, conductive gel, surrounded by an outside ring of sticky adhesive. A common use for this type of electrode is for continuous bedside monitoring.

Tab-shaped electrodes are used with 12-lead ECG monitoring and are 1½ inches long with adhesive on the long side to allow for attachment to the skin. The opposite side permits attachment of an alligator-type clip to the patient cable.

To the electrodes

TAKE HOME POINTS

Older adults may not tolerate alcohol on the skin. Sensitivity to the conductive gel on the electrode may also occur. If skin irritation is present, the electrode site should be checked and rotated every 24 hours.

Do not place electrodes in the right second intercostal space (ICS) or under the left breast. This site is used to defibrillate (electrically shock) the patient during a cardiac arrest. Shocking over an electrode will cause the force of electricity to follow the lead wires, causing damage to the patient and the equipment. It may also prevent proper voltage from being delivered to the patient. Artifact or abnormal electrical patterns on the recorded rhythm may occur if these instructions are not followed (see accompanying illustration).

What You NEED TO KNOW

Electrodes must be attached to the patient correctly to obtain a clear and accurate picture of the heart's electrical function.

What You DO

To attach electrodes to a patient, you should do the following:
- Explain what you are doing. Reassure the patient that he or she will not receive an electrical shock and that alarms do not always mean that there is a problem with his or her heartbeat.
- Provide privacy for electrode application.
- Wash your hands.
- Identify the patient by checking his or her ident-a-band and asking his or her name.
- Electrodes transmit best when they are in direct contact with skin. Avoid placing electrodes on hairy areas. Hair will interfere with contact between the skin and the electrode. Shaving is no longer an acceptable practice; it may irritate the patient's skin. Clipping the hair is preferred.
- If the skin is moist or soiled, cleanse the area with an alcohol wipe or soap and water; allow it to dry. This will remove any excess skin oils and promote good skin contact.
- Allow the area to dry thoroughly before applying the electrodes. If the patient is continuously sweating or moist (**diaphoretic**), you can apply a thin coat of a skin preparation solution and allow it to dry. However, be sure to avoid applying the solution to the area of the skin that is in direct contact with the electrode gel.

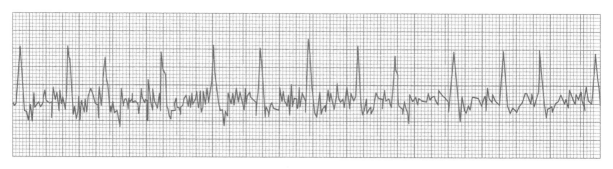

Artifact

- Keep in mind that electrodes will dry out in about 3 days, and that they should be changed every 24-48 hours per your hospital's policy.
- Avoid bony prominences. ICSs are good electrical conductors and are easy to find by palpating between the ribs.
- Avoid the ribs and sternum. Also avoid skin folds, breast tissue, and bony areas. These body areas interfere with electrical conduction and have a tendency to produce more artifact.
- Remove the electrodes from their packages.
- Snap the lead wire to the metal snap on the outside of the disc before applying. This avoids having to compress the lead wire to the electrode on the patient, which could possibly cause pain.
- Remove the paper backing from the electrode without touching the sticky adhesive. Examine the center of the disc to check if the gel is moist. If it is dry, discard and use a new disc.
- Place each electrode on the prepared site by tracing and pressing firmly around the adhesive. If your system comes with an **alligator clip** (a clip with a type of jaw attachment on the lead wire), place the tab electrode on the skin first. Squeeze the jaws of the clip open and attach it to the electrode.
- Connect the color-coded lead wires to the corresponding color on the monitor cable. For example, white lead wire goes to white monitor cable.

TAKE HOME POINTS

Placement of electrodes over large muscles may interfere with an accurate ECG analysis.

Do You UNDERSTAND?

DIRECTIONS: **Fill in the blanks.**

1. Electrical energy generated from the heart is measured in

   _____.

2. Thin, flexible wires that connect electrodes to the patient cable are called _____.

3. An _____ is a sticky pad that helps conduct electrical energy to the monitor.

4. An _____ displays waveforms of the heart's electrical activity.

DIRECTIONS: **Indicate in the spaces provided whether the following statements are *true* or *false*.**

5. _____ Bony areas increase transmission of heart impulses.

6. _____ Chest hair does not have to be removed for electrode placement.

7. _____ Large muscle groups and skin folds increase artifact.

8. _____ Electrodes should be changed every 4 to 5 days.

What IS a Lead?

A *lead* is an electrical view of the heart. Each lead represents a view from a different position. Leads consist of two *poles:* a negative pole and a positive pole. Electrical activity that flows within the heart can be recorded between the negative and positive poles (electricity flows from negative to positive).

The two poles are identified by either two electrodes, one at each pole *(bipolar)*, or they are identified as one electrode and a mathematically determined reference point *(unipolar)*. A pair of electrodes, one positive and one negative, or a single electrode and a reference point form a lead.

What You NEED TO KNOW

Normally, the electrical impulse produced in the heart starts in the sinoatrial (SA) node, which is generally located in the right upper chest. The impulse then moves toward the ventricles in the left lower chest. Therefore electrical flow is downward and to the left. This flow pattern is known as normal *axis*. **Axis** refers to the general direction of the flow of electrical activity (depolarization) as it spreads through the heart.

As the flow of electrical activity moves *from* the *negative* electrode *toward* the *positive* electrode, an upward **(positive)** wave is produced. If the flow of electrical activity moves away from the positive electrode, a downward **(negative)** wave is produced.

The camera analogy is frequently used to describe a lead **(view)**. Consider the positive electrode to be the camera lens or the recording electrode. The negative electrode would then be the director, telling the camera in which direction to shoot the picture.

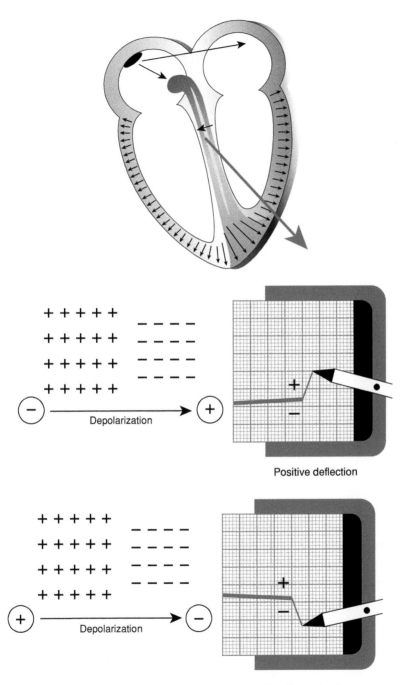

Positive deflection

Negative deflection

In addition to positive and negative electrodes, a *ground* electrode is also used. Because leakage of electricity from faulty wires can generate a shock, a *ground electrode* is needed to absorb any excess electricity. For this reason, all monitoring systems have a ground electrode and a three-pronged plug to protect the patient.

Do You UNDERSTAND?

DIRECTIONS: **Write the word or words that best define the information in each sentence.**

1. An electrode is placed at the positive pole, and a corresponding electrode is placed at the negative pole.

   _____

2. Prevents accidental shock to the patient.

   _____

3. General direction of electrical flow in the heart.

   _____

4. The direction of the deflection that will occur if the flow of electrical activity (depolarization) moves away from the positive electrode.

   _____

TAKE HOME POINTS
- To avoid confusion and misinterpretation of data, electrodes must be placed on the patient correctly.
- The flow of electrical activity in the heart does not change (the view changes with each lead).

What IS a 12-Lead ECG?

A *12-lead ECG* is a graphic display that provides 12 different, simultaneous views of the heart's electrical activity. The 12-lead ECG is used to diagnose the cause of dysrhythmia, determine conduction defects, diagnose and monitor myocardial infarction (MI), diagnose myocardial ischemia and injury, and determine cardiac position and size. It is also used to diagnose particular diseases, such as pericarditis and Wolff-Parkinson-White syndrome, and evaluate electrolyte abnormalities and the effects of drug therapy.

What You NEED TO KNOW

The heart can be viewed from four major or general surfaces. The front of the heart is considered the *anterior surface;* the back of the heart is con-

Answers: 1. bipolar; 2. ground electrode; 3. axis; 4. downward (negative).

sidered the *posterior surface;* the bottom of the heart is considered the *inferior surface;* and the left side of the heart is considered the *lateral surface.*

The 12-lead ECG can assess the electrical activity of all four surfaces of the heart. For example, if the health care provider wants to examine the anterior surface of the heart, the lead or leads that will best assess this particular heart surface are selected.

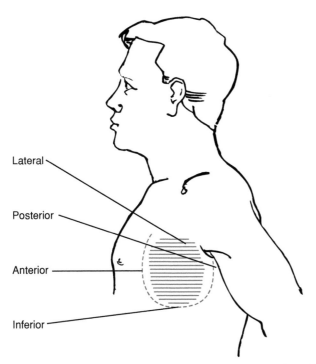

Modified from Huff: *ECG workout: exercises in arrhythmia interpretation,* ed 3, Philadelphia, 1997, Lippincott, p. 3.

The 12 leads of the ECG test are divided into two subgroups: the *limb leads,* which include standard limb leads and augmented limb leads; and the *chest leads,* known as *precordial leads* or *V leads.* Electrode placement knowledge is essential in performing a 12-lead ECG.

Four electrodes are attached to the patient's upper and lower extremities. These are the limb leads. Six electrodes are positioned in specific locations across the upper chest. These are the chest leads. Although only 10 electrode pads are attached, the ECG machine (via computer), obtains 12 views of the heart by changing poles.

LIFE SPAN

As a health-teaching tip, middle-aged and older adults should have a 12-lead ECG with their annual physical. The baseline from this test can then be used to note cardiac changes over time.

TAKE HOME POINTS

The 12-lead ECG provides multiple views of the heart's electrical activity from each of the four major heart surfaces.

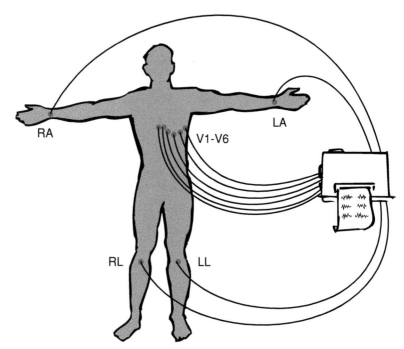

From Hudak, Gallo, Morton, editors: *Critical care nursing: a holistic approach,* ed 6, Philadelphia, 1998, Lippincott, p. 189.

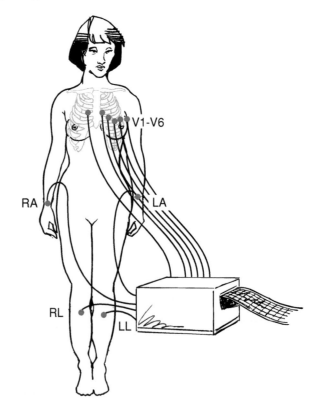

Do You UNDERSTAND?

DIRECTIONS: **Fill in the blanks.**
1. The bottom of the heart is considered the _____ surface.
2. The front of the heart is considered the _____ surface.
3. The left side of the heart is considered the _____ surface.
4. The back of the heart is considered the _____ surface.

What ARE Limb Leads?

Limb leads are the first six views of a 12-lead ECG. They are divided into *standard limb leads* and *augmented limb leads*. Limb leads record electrical activity from top to bottom and from right to left on a frontal plane of the chest. To record electrical activity from the limb leads, electrodes are placed on the right and left arms and on the left leg or foot. The placement of these electrodes forms a triangle, known as *Einthoven's triangle*. If this triangle is shortened and centered, it forms a plane over the chest. The right leg electrode may be used as a ground.

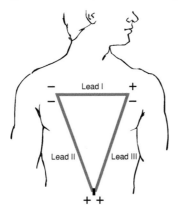

Standard Limb Leads

Standard limb leads are *bipolar*; therefore they have two electrodes: one at the positive pole and one at the negative pole. One lead wire is attached to a positive electrode on one limb, and the other is attached to a negative electrode on the other limb. Standard limb leads are designated as leads I, II, and III.

Lead I Lead I views electrical activity from the right upper chest to the left upper chest. Electrodes are placed on the right arm (negative) and the left arm (positive).

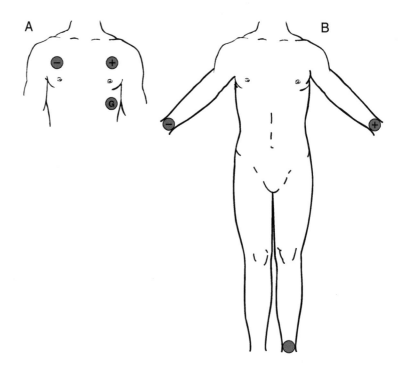

Lead II Lead II views electrical activity from the right upper chest to the left leg. Electrodes are placed on the right arm (negative) and the left leg (positive) positions.

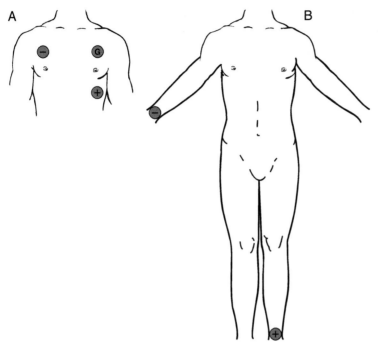

Lead III Lead III views electrical activity from the left upper chest to the left leg. Electrodes are placed on the left arm (negative) and the left leg (positive) positions.

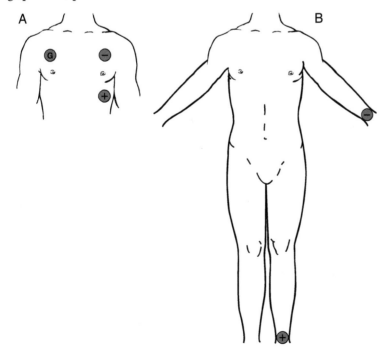

Augmented Limb Leads

Augmented limb leads are designated as *augmented voltage right arm (aVR), augmented voltage left arm (aVL),* and *augmented voltage foot (aVF).* They are called *augmented* because the voltage must be amplified 1.5-fold by the ECG machine to produce waves of the same magnitude as those of leads I, II, and III. Augmented limb leads are unipolar, because they have one positive pole and a reference point in the opposite side of the heart. However, they use the same electrode placement as the standard limb leads (right and left arm, left foot).

aVR In lead aVR, the right arm electrode is positive and the left arm and left leg electrodes are channeled together to form a common reference point that has a negative charge. In this view, the electrical wave of depolarization moves away from the positive electrode. Therefore the waveform deflections produced on the ECG paper will be downward (negative).

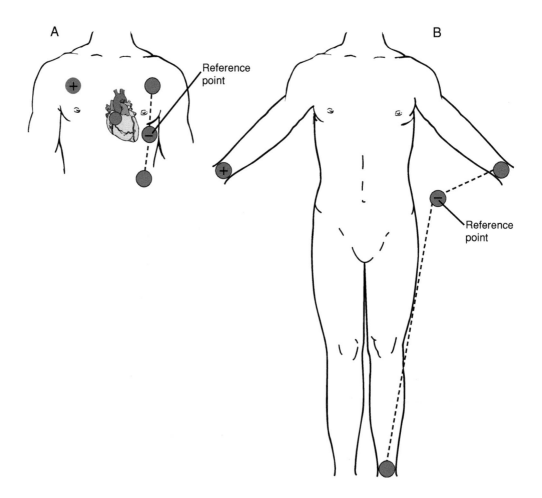

aVL In lead aVL, the left arm electrode is positive and the right arm and left leg electrodes are channeled together to form a common reference point that has a negative charge.

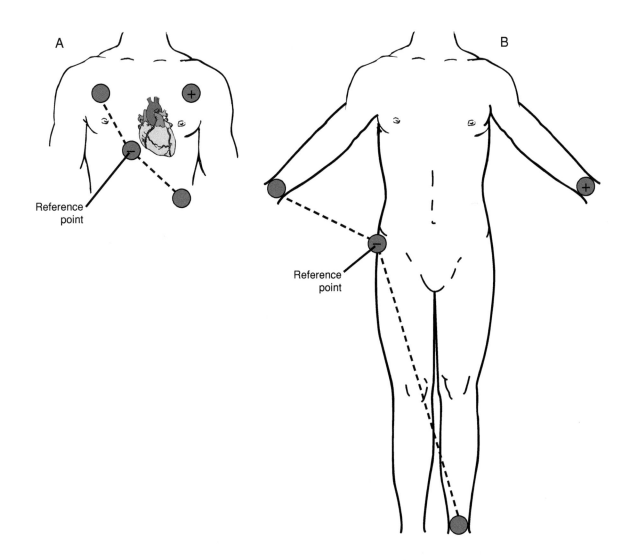

aVF In lead aVF, the left foot electrode is positive and the right arm and left arm electrodes are channeled together to form a common reference point that has a negative charge. The waveforms produced in aVF will always be upward (positive), because the general flow of electricity moves toward the positive electrode.

TAKE HOME POINTS

- The small *a* represents the word augmented.
- The *V* represents the word *voltage*.
- The *capitalized third* letter tells the health care provider where to place the positive electrode pad or tab.
- Normally, aVR produces only negative waveforms.
- Augmented leads also form intersecting lines on a plane. They view the heart from different angles than the standard leads.

What You NEED TO KNOW

The waveforms produced in the standard limb leads will always be upward (positive), because the general flow of electricity moves toward the positive electrode.

By pushing leads I, II, and III to the center of the Einthoven's triangle, three intersecting lines are formed. Each line provides a different view of the patient's chest (see accompanying illustration).

Limb leads provide views of the heart from six different angles in the *frontal plane*. This is accomplished by superimposing the intersecting lines of the standard limb leads over the intersecting lines of the augmented limb leads.

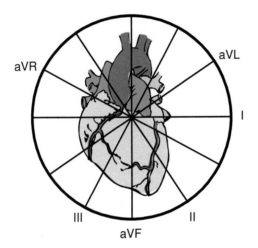

The frontal plane represents a vertical view of the heart, from superior to inferior (up to down) and from right to left.

Do You UNDERSTAND?

DIRECTIONS: **Fill in the blanks for the placement of the positive electrodes in standard and augmented leads.**

1. Lead I _____
2. Lead II _____
3. Lead III _____
4. Lead aVR _____
5. Lead aVL _____
6. Lead aVF _____

What ARE the Precordial Leads?

The last six leads of the ECG look at events in the heart on a horizontal plane. These are called the precordial, chest, or *V* leads. They are positioned directly over the heart, viewing the anterior and lateral surfaces. The positive poles are areas on the anterior and lateral chest. The negative pole is considered to be a reference point on the opposite side of the positive pole. Similar to the augmented leads, these leads are unipolar. Therefore one electrode is placed on the anterior chest (the positive electrode). To obtain the six leads, six electrodes are placed in six different positions across the anterior and lateral chest wall.

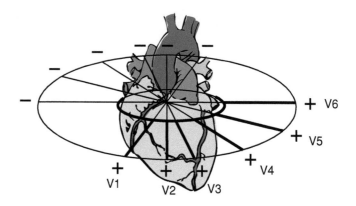

What You NEED TO KNOW

The precordial leads are placed from the right to the left of the heart. They are called *V1, V2, V3, V4, V5,* and *V6.*

V1. The positive electrode is placed directly over the right atrium. Usually, the QRS complex is negative, and the R wave is small in V1, because the flow of electricity moves away from the positive electrode.

V2. The positive electrode is placed just anterior to the atrioventricular (AV) node. Usually, the QRS complex is negative, and the R wave is slightly taller than in V1.

V3. The positive electrode is placed over the ventricular septum. The QRS complex is isoelectric, which means half is above the baseline and half is below the baseline.

V4. The positive electrode is also placed over the ventricular septum but to the left of V3. The QRS complex is more positive than in V3.

V5 and V6. The positive electrodes are placed over the lateral surface of the left ventricle. The QRS complexes are more positive than in V4.

Placement of electrodes for the precordial leads is guided by the ICSs as follows:

- **V1.** Fourth ICS, right sternal border
- **V2.** Fourth ICS, left sternal border
- **V3.** Halfway between V2 and V4
- **V4.** Fifth ICS, left midclavicular line
- **V5.** Fifth ICS, left anterior axillary line
- **V6.** Fifth ICS, left midaxillary line

The intersecting lines of the precordial leads form a horizontal plane providing six views, from anterior to posterior and from right to left. The R wave gets progressively larger from V1 to V6, as more of the ventricles are viewed. This is called *R-wave progression.*

What You DO

Correct electrode placement is crucial in obtaining the correct waveforms. To place precordial leads correctly:

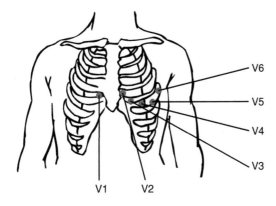

- Place the V1 electrode over the fourth ICS, to the right of the sternum.
- Place the V2 electrode just lateral to V1, at the left of the sternum at the fourth ICS.

- Skip to V4, and place the V4 electrode over the fifth ICS and mid-clavicular line or the point of maximal impulse (PMI).
- Find V3 (halfway between V2 and V4).
- Place the V6 electrode at the left midaxillary line (level with V4).
- Place the V5 electrode halfway between V4 and V6, at the anterior axillary line.

Do You UNDERSTAND?

DIRECTIONS: **Describe the location of the precordial leads.**
1. V1 _____
2. V2 _____
3. V3 _____
4. V4 _____
5. V5 _____
6. V6 _____

What You NEED TO KNOW

The 12-lead ECG takes several seconds to conduct, once you have placed the electrodes on the patient. It records the electrical activity of the heart from 12 points (6 limb leads and 6 chest leads), and documentation is provided on standard-sized paper.

This test is performed during routine physical examinations, on admission to the hospital, and when cardiac, electrical, or mechanical problems are suggested. An ECG may be prescribed by the physician or by an advanced practical nurse, or the unit may have standing orders for the provider to perform this test when the patient's condition warrants it.

Answers: 1. **Fourth ICS, to the right of the sternum;** 2. **Fourth ICS, to the left of the sternum;** 3. Find V4 first, halfway between V2 and V4; 4. **Fifth ICS, midclavicular line;** 5. Find V6 first, halfway between V4 and V6; 6. **Fifth ICS, lateral to V4, midaxillary line.**

1.

2.

3.

4.

5.

6.

What You DO

- If serial 12 leads will be obtained, it may be helpful to mark the electrode positions with permanent ink.
- Connect all cables to the designated electrodes. The patient cable is already attached to the ECG machine.
- Confirm that the 10 electrodes and cables are in the correct position.
- Enter the name, date, and patient number on the ECG.
- To avoid artifact and obtain the best quality, ask the patient to remain still during the procedure.
- Run the test according to the manufacturer's directions.

Information about the patient (name, date, time, medical record number, physician) need to be confirmed on the ECG printout. It is also important to include any symptoms that the patient may be experiencing.

TAKE HOME POINTS

Consistent placement of all electrodes is essential to detect changes in the anterior, posterior, inferior, and lateral surfaces of the heart.

Do You UNDERSTAND?

DIRECTIONS: **Indicate in the spaces provided whether the following statements are *true* or *false*.**

1. _____ The 12-lead ECG may take several hours to perform.
2. _____ To perform the 12-lead ECG, 12 electrodes are placed on various parts of the body to obtain multiple views.
3. _____ The patient should remain still while the actual ECG is being performed.

What IS Continuous ECG Monitoring?

Continuous ECG monitoring, also referred to as continuous cardiac monitoring or continuous bedside monitoring, is the continuous recording of the heart's electrical activity. Continuous ECG monitoring is mainly used to assess the heart rate, rhythm, and ST segment. Its primary function is to check for ectopy (abnormal heartbeat) or **dysrhythmia.** Continuous cardiac monitoring is accomplished using either a 3- or 5-lead system.

The 3-lead system is limited to single-channel recording, which means only one lead can be viewed on the monitor at a time. A 5-lead system allows dual-channel recording, which means that two leads can be viewed on the monitor at the same time. Continuous ECG monitoring can be accomplished either by a hardwire system (**bedside monitoring**) or by telemetry. Continuous ECG monitoring by telemetry uses radio waves rather than electricity to deliver information about the heart's electrical activity to a monitor.

What You NEED TO KNOW

With continuous monitoring, the limb leads are placed on the chest, not on the limbs as in standard 12-lead ECG monitoring. Arm leads should be placed on the shoulders, close to where the limbs join the body. The right arm *(RA)* is placed in the right shoulder area, and the left arm *(LA)* is placed in the left shoulder area. The right leg *(RL)* is moved up to the right abdominal area, and the left leg *(LL)* is moved up to the left abdominal area.

Hardwire or Bedside Monitoring

Continuous ECG monitoring or *bedside cardiac monitoring* by *hardwire* requires the patient to be directly connected to a large monitoring device at the bedside. This system is used when patients are limited to bedrest, and it operates on electricity. Information is transmitted to the bedside monitor via lead wires and cables and to the central station by hardwire (electrically). There are many settings in which this type of monitoring is used, including intensive care units (ICUs), emergency departments (EDs), operating rooms (ORs), day surgery centers, and cardiac catheterization laboratories.

Telemetry

Telemetry is accomplished by using short cables, which are connected to a small, portable radio transmitter. The heart's electrical activity is transmitted by radio waves from the transmitter to ceiling antennas. This information is then transmitted to a central monitoring station. The transmitter is battery powered and can be carried by the patient in a pocket or pouch, allowing the patient to freely move around. Telemetry monitoring is used on units where patients no longer require intensive care but still require close cardiac surveillance.

 Cellular phones can disrupt the transmission of radio waves. Therefore the use of cellular phones is not permitted on or near telemetry units.

What IS a 3-Lead System?

A *3-lead* or *3-electrode system* is a continuous monitoring system with three patient wires. These electrode systems are the easiest to learn and are used wherever quick monitoring is needed (in EDs, telemetry units, and first responder units). The advantage of the 3-lead system is that it is less expensive and requires less memory than other systems, because only three electrodes and three patient lead wires are required. This system is limited to single-channel (one lead) viewing.

What You NEED TO KNOW

The standard placement for electrodes in a 3-lead system are on the right shoulder area under the clavicle and on the left shoulder area under the clavicle on the lower left chest area, below the fifth ICS or apex of the heart. The three leads are color-coded white, black, and red.

What You DO

The color-coded leads are connected as follows:
- The white lead wire, designated RA, is attached to the right arm electrode.
- The black lead wire, designated LA, is attached to the left arm electrode.
- The red lead wire, designated LL, is attached to the electrode on the left lower chest.

   With this pattern of electrode placement, the 3-lead system can be used to monitor the standard limb leads I, II, or III by turning the selector dial. *No* electrodes need to be moved. The selector on the monitoring device automatically adjusts, determining which electrode will be positive, which will be negative, and which will be the ground, depending on the lead view selected.

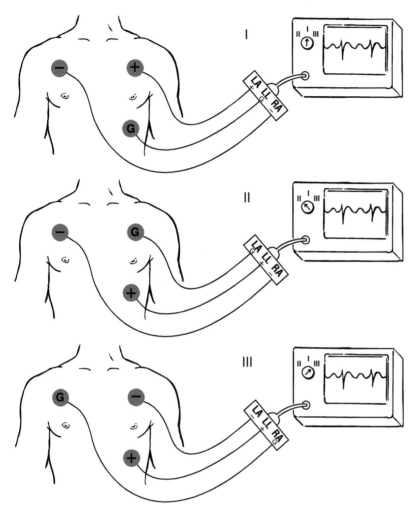

Standard Lead Placement in a 3-Lead System

Lead	Positive	Negative	Ground
Lead I	Left arm	Right arm	Left lower chest
Lead II	Left lower chest	Right arm	Left arm
Lead III	Left lower chest	Left arm	Right arm

 TAKE HOME POINTS

- The left lower electrode must be placed below the level of the heart.
- To recall lead placement for the 3-lead system, remember "white is right" and "smoke over fire." The white lead goes on the right arm, and the black lead goes over the red lead on the left.
- Lead I is useful for patients with respiratory distress, because chest wall motion is least affected in this lead.
- Lead II is preferred for observing the patient's underlying rhythm, because lead II produces the most upright waveforms. Lead II is a primary monitoring lead for dysrhythmia detection.

A patient may need to receive defibrillation. If defibrillator pads are placed over electrodes, the electricity produced from defibrillation will travel through the lead wires and electrodes and could cause harm to the patient and equipment. When placing electrodes on a patient, avoid the apex of the heart to ensure that the defibrillator pads fit in these areas.

What IS a Modified Chest Lead (MCL)?

Frequently, it is necessary to record electrical activity from the heart's anterior or lateral surface to assess ventricular rhythm disturbances.

Modified chest lead 1 (MCL1) and modified chest lead 6 (MCL6) are useful for identifying bundle branch blocks and for differentiating supraventricular tachycardia from ventricular tachycardia.

What You NEED TO KNOW

Lead MCL1 is the modified version of the precordial lead V1. Lead MCL6 is the modified version of the precordial lead V6. To obtain these views with a 3-lead system, you must move the electrodes.

From Hudak, Gallo, Morton, editors: *Critical care nursing: a holistic approach,* ed 6, Philadelphia, 1998, Lippincott, p. 203.

What You DO

To use MCL1 and MCL6 to record electrical activity from the heart's anterior or lateral surface:

- Connect one electrode to the *LA* lead wire, and place it in the V1 position. This becomes the positive electrode.
- Connect one electrode to the *RA* lead wire, and place it in the left arm position. This becomes the negative electrode.
- Connect one electrode to the *LL* lead wire, and place it in the V6 position. This becomes the ground electrode.
- Turn the monitor's selector dial to lead 1.

Obtain a 12-lead ECG to confirm any significant rhythm disturbances. Remember, it is the correct attachment to the correct color and the proper placement of electrodes that determine the accuracy of the ECG waveform.

Once these electrodes are in place, you may also monitor the lateral surface lead MCL6. To obtain a lateral surface view, turn the selector dial to lead II.

Do You UNDERSTAND?

DIRECTIONS: On the diagrams that follow, label the negative, positive, and ground electrode placement for leads II and MCL1.

1. Lead II

2. Lead MCL

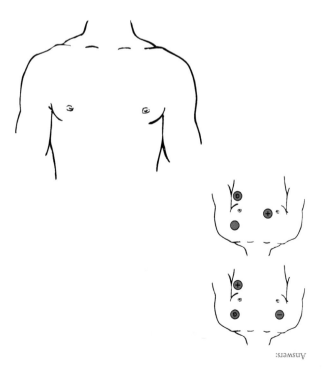

Answers:

What IS a 5-Lead System?

A *5-lead system* is used in recovery rooms, intensive care units, EDs, and telemetry units. This system includes five electrodes and five lead wires that attach to a patient cable, and it allows for continuous monitoring of the patient's electrical heart rhythm in two *leads* or lead views at the same time (*dual lead* monitoring).

What You NEED TO KNOW

The 5-lead system adds a right leg *(RL)* and a chest electrode *(V1 position)* to the previous 3-lead standard electrode placement. By adding the *RL* electrode, any of the six limb leads can be viewed. The *chest* electrode can be moved to any of the precordial *V* positions to obtain all six precordial views. Review the sections on limb leads and precordial leads.

TAKE HOME POINTS

The 5-lead system can provide all 12 views of the 12-lead ECG, but not simultaneously. Additionally, it requires that the chest electrode be moved to obtain any of the V-lead position views.

To confirm and document a dysrhythmia before starting treatment, the use of more than one lead may be necessary.

In the 5-lead system, leads II and V1 are used the most.

What You DO

In a 5-lead system:
- Two electrodes are placed in the right and left second ICS spaces, at the midclavicular lines.
- Two are placed at the right and left seventh ICS spaces, at the midaxillary line.
- The chest electrode is placed at the fourth ICS space to the right of the sternum.

Do You UNDERSTAND?

DIRECTIONS: List the advantages of a 3-lead system and a 5-lead system.

Advantages of a 3-lead system

1. _____

2. _____

3. _____

Advantages of a 5-lead system

4. _____

5. _____

6. _____

TAKE HOME POINTS
- Color-coded lead wire system
  Right upper arm = white
  Left upper arm = black
  Right fourth ICS = brown
  Right lower chest = green
  Left lower chest = red
- The monitor internally changes the designation of positive and negative electrodes when you turn the selector dial to a specific lead.

Examine lead wires, patient cables, and monitors for loose connections and physical damage to avoid potential electrical shock to the patient.

Answers: **1. Easy to apply; 2. Quick; 3. Patient freedom; 4. Dual-lead monitoring; 5. No need to move electrodes for most leads; 6. Allows all views of a 12-lead ECG.**

DIRECTIONS: **Write the placement and color of the electrodes in a 5-lead monitoring system on the following illustration of the patient's torso.**

What IS Selection of a Monitoring Lead?

Systems monitor and record the patient's heart rhythm in more than one view at the same time. You will need to select a monitoring lead, based on your patient's needs, which will be different from patient to patient, depending on the patient's cardiac status.

What You NEED TO KNOW

Lead II remains the preferred lead for monitoring a patient's underlying rhythm. V1 or MCL1 and V6 or MCL6 are preferred for identifying bundle branch blocks and ventricular ectopy. See the following table for suggested monitoring lead selection.

Answers:

Suggested Monitoring Lead Selection

Lead	Rationale for Use
II	Produces large, upright visible P waves and QRS complexes for determining underlying rhythm
V1 or MCL1	Helpful for detecting right bundle branch block and for differentiating ventricular ectopy from supraventricular rhythms and aberrant conduction in the ventricles
V6 or MCL6	Helpful lead for detecting left bundle branch block for differentiating ventricular ectopy from supraventricular rhythm aberrantly conducted in the ventricles
III, aVF, V1	Produce visible P waves; useful in detecting atrial dysrhythmias; useful in patients with respiratory distress; involved left- and right-arm electrode placements are less affected by chest motion compared with other leads
II, III, aVF	Helpful in detecting ischemia, injury, and infarction in the inferior wall
I, aVL, V5, V6	Helpful in detecting ischemia, injury, and infarction in the lateral wall
V1 through V4	Helpful in detecting ischemia, injury, and infarction in the anterior wall

Vectorcardiography

Newer 5-lead systems have the capability of monitoring 12-leads simultaneously. Conventional ECGs provide flat, frontal, and horizontal views. However, Dr. E. Frank developed *vectorcardiography* to obtain three-dimensional (3-D) views.

The 3-D views are obtained in the following way:
- Frontal plane—right to left (X) and head to foot (Y)
- Horizontal plane—right to left (X) and anterior to posterior (Z)
- Sagittal plane—head to foot (Y) and anterior to posterior (Z)

To obtain multiple 3-D views, Dr. E. Frank developed an 8-electrode placement system. This system has been modified to perform 12-lead ECG monitoring with a 5-lead continuous monitoring system. A 5-lead continuous monitoring system can derive a 12-lead ECG by using three of Frank's electrode sites: *E, A,* and *I.* An *S* site is added to the upper sternum, and a ground is added to the right lower area. This is called the *EASI method.*

Redrawn from Franks: *3D view of the heart; application note, 12-lead monitoring with EASI lead system,* 1999, Agilent Technologies.

Redrawn from Franks: *3D view of the heart; application note, 12-lead monitoring with EASI lead system,* 1999, Agilent Technologies.

TAKE HOME POINTS

Because the entire medical community has not accepted this new technology, the 12-lead ECG remains the *gold standard* for ECG monitoring.

Redrawn from Franks: *3D view of the heart; application note, 12-lead monitoring with EASI lead system*, 1999, Agilent Technologies.

Do You UNDERSTAND?

DIRECTIONS: **Indicate in the spaces provided whether the following statements are *true* or *false*.**

1. _____ Newer 5-lead continuous-monitoring systems have the capability to perform a 12-lead ECG.

2. _____ With the EASI method of electrode placement, the S electrode is placed in the V1 position.

3. _____ Vectorcardiography views the heart in three dimensions, rather than on planes as in standard 12-lead monitoring.

References

About Nursing: How to apply cardiac monitoring electrodes in a 5-leadwire system. Available at nursing.about.com/cs/aclsblsekg/ht/applyelectrodes.htm.

Agilent Technologies: *12-lead monitoring with EASI lead system, App Note,* Palo Alto, CA, 1999, Agilent Technologies.

Boyer MJ: *Lippincott's need-to-know ECG facts,* Philadelphia, 1997, Lippincott.

Dubin D: *Rapid interpretation of EKGs,* ed 5, Tampa, FL, 1996, Cover Publishing.

Ehrat KS: *The art of EKG interpretation: a self-instructional text,* ed 4, Dubuque, IA, 1997, Kendall/Hunt.

Huff J: *ECG workout: exercises in arrhythmia interpretation,* ed 3, Philadelphia, 1997, Lippincott.

Jacobson C: Advanced ECG concepts. In Chulay M, Gizzetta C, and Dossey B, editors: *AACN handbook of critical care nursing,* Stamford, CT, 1997, Appleton & Lange.

Johns C: Nursing management of arrhythmias. In Lewis SM, Heitkemper HH, Dirksen SR, editors: *Medical-surgical nursing,* ed 5, St Louis, 2000, Mosby.

Lewis KM: *Sensible ECG analysis,* Albany, NY, 2000, Delmar Publishing.

Lewis SM, Heitkemper HH, Dirksen SR: *Medical-surgical nursing,* ed 5, St Louis, 2000, Mosby.

McAvoy J: Case studies of ST-segment elevation before and after percutaneous coronary intervention in patients with acute myocardial infarction, *Crit Care Nurse* 24(6):32-39, 2004.

McHale JD, Carlson KK: *AACN procedure manual for critical care,* ed 4, Philadelphia, 2001, Saunders.

Paul S, Hebra J: *The nurse's guide to cardiac rhythm interpretation: implications for patient care,* Philadelphia, 1998, Saunders.

Woods S: Dysrhythmia interpretation. In Sole LS, Lamborn ML, Hartshorn JC, editors: *Introduction to critical care nursing,* ed 3, Philadelphia, 2001, Saunders.

Answers: **1. True; 2. False; 3. True.**

NCLEX® Review

1. Provider Jones has worked in the coronary care unit for 6 years and is overseeing the training of Ms. Confer, GN. Provider Jones knows Ms. Confer understands the rationale for a ground electrode when she states:
   1 "The ground electrode magnifies the lead of the heart so that the nurse can see it."
   2 "The ground electrode changes the lead of the heart."
   3 "The ground electrode prevents electrical shock to the patient."
   4 "The ground electrode records the current of electricity, from positive to negative."

2. Which of the following best describes lead II?
   1 Negative on the right arm, positive on the left arm
   2 Negative on the left arm, positive on the right arm
   3 Negative on the right arm, positive on the left lower chest
   4 Negative on the left arm, positive on the left lower chest

3. A 12-lead ECG is being recorded by an unlicensed assistive person. The waveform looks unusual in aVR. The registered nurse knows that the proper placement of electrodes for aVR is:
   1 Left arm positive, heart negative
   2 Right arm positive, negative reference point
   3 Right leg positive, negative reference point
   4 Right arm negative, left leg positive

4. The health care provider is performing a 12-lead ECG on a patient. The patient asks the provider to explain why so many electrodes are needed across the chest. Which of the following is the best explanation for this patient?
   1 Electrode placement across the chest ensures accuracy of heart conduction.
   2 The six sticky tabs across your chest look at the heart from top to bottom.

3 These electrodes are needed to look at your heart in the frontal plane.
4 These electrodes will tell me about your heart, from right to left.

NCLEX® Review Answers

1. **3** A ground wire prevents leakage of current and electrical shock. The augmented leads magnify the view of the heart. The placement of the positive and negative electrodes changes the lead. The axis of the lead describes where the flow of energy goes.

2. **3** In lead II, the negative electrode is on the right shoulder and the positive electrode is on the left lower chest area. "Negative on the right arm, positive on the left arm" describes lead I. "Negative left arm and positive right arm" does not describe any lead. "Negative left arm and positive left lower chest" describes lead III.

3. **2** The augmented leads are unipolar with only one electrode. This single electrode is positive. The heart surface itself provides the negative pole. The placement of the positive electrode is identified by the last letter in the lead's abbreviation. In aV*R*, the *R*ight arm is positive with a negative reference point opposite. In aV*F*, the left leg (*F*oot) is positive with a negative reference point opposite. In aV*L*, the *L*eft arm is positive with a negative reference point opposite.

4. **4** The electrode placement in the V leads looks at the heart from right ventricle (V1) to left ventricle (V6). Electrode placement across the chest ensures accuracy of heart conduction and describes the V leads, but it does not state why or answer the patient's questions. The leads do not look at the heart from top to bottom; they look at it from right to left. The V leads look at the heart in the horizontal plane.

Normal Sinus Rhythm

What You WILL LEARN

After reading this chapter, you will know how to do the following:

✔ Define normal sinus rhythm (NSR).

✔ List the names of the two waves and one complex associated with NSR.

What IS Normal Sinus Rhythm?

Normal sinus rhythm (NSR) represents the normal electrical activity of the heart. A normal heartbeat occurs when an electrical impulse is generated in the sinoatrial (SA) node in the heart. This impulse is normally generated between 60 and 100 times per minute. This electrical impulse travels from the SA node and throughout the conduction system *(review Conduction System in Chapter 1)*, causing depolarization and repolarization of both atria and both ventricles *(review Depolarization and Repolarization in Chapter 2)*. It is the electrical events of depolarization and repolarization that are seen on the electrocardiogram (ECG) paper. Depolarization of both atria produces a P wave on the ECG paper. This is followed by depolarization of both ventricles, which produces the QRS complex on the ECG paper. Repolarization of both atria occurs at the same time that the ventricles are depolarizing and therefore cannot be captured on the ECG paper. The last wave seen is the T wave, which represents ventricular repolarization completing one electrical cardiac cycle. After a short pause, the SA node generates another electrical impulse, and the cardiac cycle repeats itself, and so on, producing a regular sinus rhythm (RSR) or normal sinus rhythm (NSR).

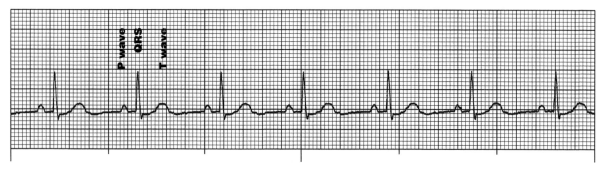

From Aehlert: *ECGs made easy,* ed 2, St Louis, 2001, Mosby, p. 74.

What You NEED TO KNOW

Normally, pacemaker cells within the SA node spontaneously depolarize faster than other cardiac cells, thus making the SA node the dominant "pacemaker of the heart." Once this electrical impulse begins, it continues its transmission via the conduction system to transitional cells at the periphery of the SA node, continuing to the myocardial cells of the surrounding atria, AV junction, bundle branches, and then to the ventricular, Purkinje muscle fibers. If the SA node fails as pacemaker of the heart, the AV can take over as pacemaker. The AV node generates impulses at a rate of 40 to 60 times per minute. If both the SA node and AV node fail as pacemakers, the Purkinje fibers in the ventricles can take over as pacemaker. The Purkinje fibers in the ventricles fire at a rate of 20 to 40 times per minute.

An NSR is characterized by a regular atrial and ventricular rate of depolarization with one positive P wave preceding each QRS complex. All P waves are uniform in appearance, and each PR interval measures 0.12 to 0.20 seconds. The duration of each QRS complex measures 0.11 seconds or less.

TAKE HOME POINTS

An ECG does NOT show mechanical events (contraction) of the heart but rather electrical activity. In NSR, however, coupling of electrical and mechanical events are assumed.

Characteristics of NSR

* Rate: 60-100 beats per minute (bpm).
* Rhythm: Regular.
* P wave: Both atria depolarize and are uniform, upright (positive) in lead II; one precedes each QRS complex.
* PR interval: 0.12 to 0.20 seconds, constant from beat to beat.
* QRS duration: Less than or equal to 0.10 seconds.

Variations in electrical impulses of the heart can occur and are collectively called dysrhythmias (also previously called arrhythmias). The variations may occur in rate (i.e., slow versus fast) and/or in rhythm (pattern or regularity).

TAKE HOME POINTS

A dysrhythmia is abnormal electrical activity within the heart, usually caused by medications, diseases, or conditions (i.e., endotracheal suctioning).

What You DO

Assess each ECG to see if it is in NSR. See the ECG below.

1. Is the rhythm regular? If the rhythm is regular, the P-P interval and the R-R intervals will be consistent.
2. Is the ventricular rate between 60 and 100 beats per minute (bpm)?

3. Is each P wave small and rounded and preceding each QRS complex?
4. Is the PR interval (time it takes the electrical impulse to travel from the SA node to the ventricles) between 0.12 and 0.20 seconds? Note that the PR interval is measured from the beginning of the P wave to the beginning of the QRS complex.
5. Is the QRS complex duration less than or equal to 0.11 seconds?

TAKE HOME POINTS

If the answer is "yes" to all of these questions, the patient is in an NSR. If the answer is "no" to any of these questions, the patient is not in an NSR.

From Aehlert: *ECGs made easy,* ed 2, St Louis, 2001, Mosby, p. 74.

Patients with NSR may develop clinically significant cardiac events.

Although a patient has a normal electrocardiogram, he/she is not necessarily healthy nor without comorbid diseases. For example, a patient with heart failure can be successfully treated with the medication digitalis with his ECG showing NSR. Another patient can have NSR and have moderate mitral valve regurgitation. There is current research investigating NSR with heart rate variability (HRV) and its relationship to cardiac function and disease/conditions, such as sleep apnea and mitral valve prolapse.

Example

Assess this ECG, and determine if it represents NSR.

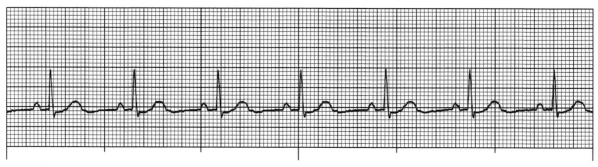

From Aehlert: *ECGs made easy,* ed 2, St Louis, 2001, Mosby, p. 74.

Answer to Example

Rhythm is regular; the rate is between 60 and 100 bpm; P waves are small and rounded and precede each QRS complex; PR interval is between 0.12 and 0.20 seconds; QRS complexes are less than or equal to 0.10 seconds. This is NSR.

Do You UNDERSTAND?

DIRECTIONS: **Read the following 10 ECGs and determine if they represent NSR. If they do not, state why.**

1.

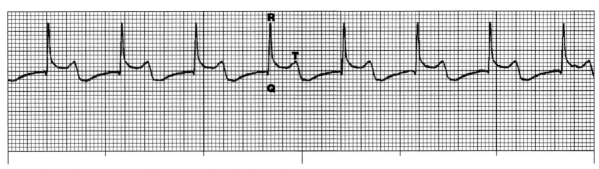

From Aehlert: *ECGs made easy,* ed 2, St Louis, 2001, Mosby, p. 261.

2.

From Aehlert: *ECGs made easy,* ed 2, St Louis, 2001, Mosby, p. 86.

3.

From Aehlert: *ECGs made easy,* ed 2, St Louis, 2001, Mosby, p. 260.

Answers: 1, Not NSR, P wave missing; 2, NSR; 3, Not NSR, PR interval too long.

4.

From Aehlert: *ECGs made easy,* ed 2, St Louis, 2001, Mosby, p. 84.

5.

From Aehlert: *ECGs made easy,* ed 2, St Louis, 2001, Mosby, p. 84.

6.

From Aehlert: *ECGs made easy,* ed 2, St Louis, 2001, Mosby, p. 84.

Answers: 4, Not NSR, rate less than 60 bpm; 5, Not NSR, QRS complex too wide; 6, NSR.

7.

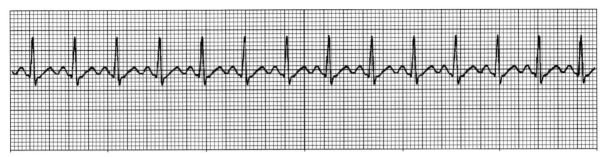

From Aehlert: *ECGs made easy,* ed 2, St Louis, 2001, Mosby, p. 85.

8.

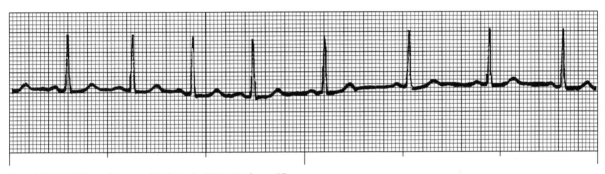

From Aehlert: *ECGs made easy,* ed 2, St Louis, 2001, Mosby, p. 87.

9.

From Aehlert: *ECGs made easy,* ed 2, St Louis, 2001, Mosby, p. 86.

Answers: 7, Not NSR, rate greater than 100 bpm; 8, Not NSR, rhythm irregular; 9, NSR.

10.

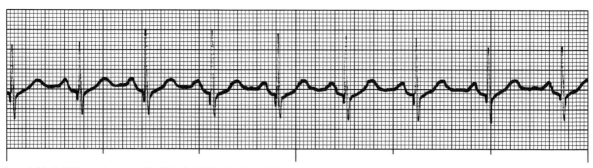

From Aehlert: *ECGs made easy,* ed 2, St Louis, 2001, Mosby, p. 85.

References

Elijah RF et al: Doppler correlation of pulmonary versus flow patterns to mitral valve regurgitant severity in patients with atrial fibrillation, *Journal of Diagnostic Medical Sonography* 14(1):4-8, 1998.

Zywietz CW et al: ECG analysis for sleep apnea detection, *Methods Inf Med* 43(1):56-59, 2004.

NCLEX® Review

1. Normal sinus rhythm (NSR) represents:
   1 Oxygenation impulses between the lungs and heart.
   2 Degree of strength of the contraction of heart muscle tissue.
   ③ Electrical activity of the heart.
   4 Complete inactivity of the nares.

2. In a normal heart beat the electrical impulse is originally started in the:
   1 Bundle of His.
   ② Sinoatrial (SA) node.
   3 Atrioventricular (AV) node.
   4 Purkinje fibers.

3. The P wave on an electrocardiogram represents:
   1 Ventricular repolarization.
   2 Depolarization of both ventricles.
   3 Repolarization of the bundle of His.
   ④ Depolarization of both atria.

4. Which of the following waves and complexes represent NSR?
   1 P wave followed by T wave then QRS complex
   ② P wave followed by QRS complex then T wave
   3 QRS complex followed by P wave then T wave
   4 T wave followed by QRS complex then ventricular repolarization

5. If the SA node fails as the pacemaker, what area of the heart takes over next as the pacemaker?
   ① AV node
   2 Purkinje fibers
   3 Bundle of His
   4 Mitral valve

6. The AV node generates an impulse rate of how many beats per minute (bpm)?
   1 60-80
   ② 40-60
   3 20-30

4 10-20

7. Variations in electrical impulses of the heart are collectively called:
   1 Interval dysfunctions
   2 Irregular spikes
   3 Rate pattern impulses (RPIs)
   ④ Dysrhythmias

8. Which of the following statements represents NSR?
   1 For every QRS complex there are two P waves.
   2 Each QRS complex duration is greater than 0.3 seconds.
   3 Each P wave is small and rounded.
   4 Ventricular rate is between 20 and 40 bpm.

NCLEX® Review Answers

1. 3 Answers 1 and 2 are wrong because ECG represents electrical activity, not oxygenation or contraction of heart muscle. Answer 4 is wrong because the nares are the nostrils in your nose and have no connection to an ECG.

2. 2 The succession of pacemaker activity is SA node, then AV node, then Purkinje fibers.

3. 4 The T wave represents ventricular repolarization, the QRS complex represents depolarization of both ventricles, and there is no ECG reading for repolarization of the bundle of His.

4. 2 NSR begins with a P wave (depolarization of both atria), followed by the QRS complex (depolarization of both ventricles), then the T wave (ventricular repolarization). Repolarization of the atria occurs at the same time the ventricles are depolarizing and therefore is not captured on an ECG.

5. 1 The succession of pacemaker activity is SA node, then AV node, then Purkinje fibers. The mitral valve has no pacemaker activity.

6. 2 Ventricular rate is 40-60 bpm.

7. 4 Answers 1, 2, and 3 are made up words.

8. 3 Answer 1 is wrong because there should be one P wave for every QRS. Answer 2 is wrong because QRS <0.10 seconds. Answer 4 is wrong because ventricular rate is 40-60 bpm.

Notes

Chapter 8
Practice Strips

Please analyze and identify information for each of the following ECG strips.

Strip 1   Rate: _____   Rhythm: _____   P wave: _____

PR interval: _____   QRS: _____

Rhythm interpretation: _____

Strip 2   Rate: _____   Rhythm: _____   P wave: _____

PR interval: _____   QRS: _____

Rhythm interpretation: _____

Strip 3   Rate: _____   Rhythm: _____   P wave: _____

PR interval: _____   QRS: _____

Rhythm interpretation: _____

Sinus Dysrhythmias: Rhythms of the Sinoatrial Node

What You WILL LEARN

After reading this chapter, you will know how to do the following:
- ✔ State the purpose of the sinoatrial node.
- ✔ Define sinus tachycardia.
- ✔ Define sinus bradycardia.
- ✔ Name two types of sinus dysrhythmias.
- ✔ Describe sinoatrial arrest or block.

What IS the Sinoatrial Node?

The *sinoatrial* (SA) *node* is the normal pacemaker of the heart. It consists of a small group of cardiac cells that generate an electrical impulse. This impulse is conducted down the normal conduction pathway, causing depolarization of the heart, which is normally followed by contraction (see Chapter 1). The SA node initiates this pacing impulse at a regular rate of 60 to 100 beats per minute (bpm). At rest, this rate is constant and unvarying, thereby producing cycles of equal length called a *regular rhythm*.

What You NEED TO KNOW

SA node stimulation results in the following:

- Regular rate of 60 to 100 bpm, with a regular rhythm
- Electrocardiogram (ECG) that shows uniform (consistent in shape) P waves
- Constant PR interval of 0.12 to 0.20 seconds
- Uniform QRS complexes of 0.04 to 0.11 seconds
- Constant QT intervals

This physiologic pattern of heart rhythm produced by the SA node is considered normal and therefore called *normal sinus rhythm* (NSR).

Basically, the heart conduction system begins at the SA node and travels through atrial tissue to the atrioventricular (AV) node. It then travels to the bundle of His, through the Purkinje fibers, and to the ventricular tissue. Any change or disturbance in the heart's conduction system (or from NSR) is called either an abnormal heart rhythm (**cardiac dysrhythmia**) or abnormal heart beat (**cardiac ectopy**).

> **TAKE HOME POINTS**
>
> Although all cardiac cells have the ability to initiate a heartbeat, the SA node provides the best physiologic rate and rhythm to sustain adequate cardiac output. The SA node is therefore considered the *"Master Pacemaker."*

> **TAKE HOME POINTS**
>
> NSR is the rhythm with which all the dysrhythmias are compared.
>
> **Criteria for identifying normal sinus rhythm**
> - **P waves:** Rounded and consistent in shape; one in front of every QRS complex
> - **Rate:** Between 60 and 100 bpm
> - **Rhythm:** Regular
> - **PR intervals:** 0.12 to 0.20 seconds
> - **QRS complex:** 0.04 to 0.11 seconds
> - **QT interval:** 0.36 to 0.44 seconds

Dysrhythmia

A *dysrhythmia* of the SA node primarily results from overactivity of either the sympathetic nervous system (SNS) or the parasympathetic nervous system (PNS). Damage to the SA node after a heart attack or administration of certain drugs (epinephrine) may also influence sinus node functioning.

Now let us examine various dysrhythmias of the SA node in detail to learn about their characteristics, causes, treatments, expected outcomes, and complications.

What You DO

- Assess the previous ECG strip for uniformity in the P wave, PR interval, and QRS complexes.
- Determine atrial and ventricular rates.
- Identify whether the rhythm is regular or irregular by measuring the distances between the R waves. If the distances are equal, the rhythm is regular.
- Essentially, you are assessing the ECG strip for NSR.
- Assess patient health factors that may cause changes in the heart's conduction (e.g., heart disease, thyroid disease, noncompliance with medications, use of illicit drugs).

Sinus dysrhythmia occurs more commonly in children and adolescents. Bradycardia can occur postoperatively in children because of inflammation or permanent injury of the SA node. They are, however, often asymptomatic because they can increase their stroke volumes and maintain their cardiac outputs. Bradycardia, sinus arrest, or sinus block may occur in older adults, because long-term hypertension or atherosclerosis affects the blood supply to the SA node.

Do You UNDERSTAND?

DIRECTIONS: **Number the components of heart conduction in the correct sequence.**

1. __D__ a. AV node
   __b__ b. Atrial tissue
   __a__ c. Purkinje fibers
   __e__ d. SA node
   __c__ e. Bundle of His
   __f__ f. Ventricular tissue

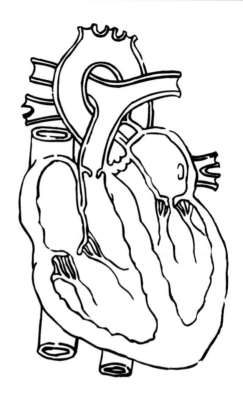

DIRECTIONS: **Use different colored pens or pencils to trace the components of conduction.**

2. a. SA node to AV node
   b. AV node to Purkinje fibers

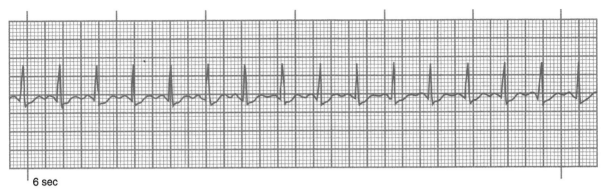

6 sec

Redrawn from Cohn, Gilroy-Doohan: *Flip and see ECG,* Philadelphia, 1996, Saunders, p. 77.

What IS Sinus Tachycardia?

A *sinus tachycardia* occurs when the SA node discharges impulses at a rate of 101 to 150 impulses per minute and when each impulse is conducted through the normal conduction pathway, followed by contraction. Sinus tachycardia, therefore, follows all the same criteria of the NSR, *except for the rate* of 101 to 150 bpm.

What You NEED TO KNOW

The patient may report a sensation of rapid heartbeat (palpitations), complain of dizziness, or become short of breath. These symptoms occur because the rapid rate decreases ventricular filling time, causing a decreased stroke volume and lower blood pressure, which results in a reduction of cardiac output and inadequate tissue perfusion. Thus, less blood will be available to the body for its use.

Sinus tachycardia is most commonly caused by SNS stimulation (the fight-or-flight response). It may be triggered by fear, anxiety, exercise, excitement, pain, some drugs, fever, hypovolemic shock (from bleeding or dehydration), or heart failure.

In a person with cardiac disease, this rapid heart rate could trigger congestive heart failure or a heart attack, if the cardiac muscle is unable to sustain the rapid rate. In these cases, medication to slow the rate is indicated.

What You DO

If you suspect that a patient has sinus tachycardia, you should:

- Treat the underlying cause. For example, identify and control the source of fear, anxiety, or pain to reduce or eliminate the source of the fight-or-flight response; give antipyretics as prescribed to reduce fever; identify the drug source for which sympathetic stimulation is a known side effect, such as aminophylline. Sinus tachycardia is usually not treated with heart medication.
- Once the underlying cause is identified and removed, the heart rate will return to normal, and, if experienced, palpitations, shortness of breath (**dyspnea**), and dizziness should subside. In the person with an otherwise normal heart, no complications should arise.
- Identify the rapid rate as sinus tachycardia, and document it.
- Consider possible causes most applicable to the patient's unique situation; investigate further through collection of subjective and objective data, and share results with the primary care provider.
- Be alert for signs and symptoms heralding other problems, such as lack of perfusion caused by inadequate blood volume (**hypovolemic shock**) that results in restlessness; decreased blood pressure; pallor; thirst; weak pulse; or early heart failure, resulting in restlessness and the need to sit up to breathe easier (**orthopnea**) or to cough.

TAKE HOME POINTS

To determine whether a rhythm is sinus tachycardia, observe for the following:

- **Rate:** A rapid heart rate is between 101 and 150 bpm.
- **Rhythm:** Regular; P-P intervals and R-R intervals are equal.
- **P wave:** P wave should be uniform in shape and present before each QRS complex.
- **QRS:** QRS complexes should look alike and be 0.04 to 0.11 seconds apart.
- **PR interval:** The interval is between 0.12 and 0.20 seconds.

Do You UNDERSTAND?

DIRECTIONS: **Place a check by the characteristics, causes, or treatments that apply to sinus tachycardia.**

1. _____ a. Rate less than 60 bpm
   __✓__ b. Rate greater than 100 bpm
   __✓__ c. Results from SNS stimulation
   _____ d. Results from PNS stimulation
   _____ e. Results in irregularities in waveforms and rhythms
   __✓__ f. Waveforms and rhythms remain regular
   __✓__ g. Caused by fear, anxiety, pain
   _____ h. Caused by medications, such as sympathetic blockers
   _____ i. First, give medications to reduce the rate
   __✓__ j. Identify underlying cause and attempt to treat it

Answers: 1. b, c, f, g, j.

DIRECTIONS: **Indicate in the spaces provided whether the following statements related to sinus tachycardia are *true* or *false*.**

2. _____ Sinus tachycardia decreases the workload of the heart.
3. _____ The first intervention for sinus tachycardia is an appropriate drug.
4. _____ Sinus tachycardia can be initiated by physical or emotional causes.
5. _____ Sinus tachycardia can be a sign of more serious health problems, such as hemorrhage or heart failure.

DIRECTIONS: **The following strip is an example of sinus tachycardia. Prove this by comparing it with the information in the previous "Take Home Points" section. Place your findings on the spaces provided.**

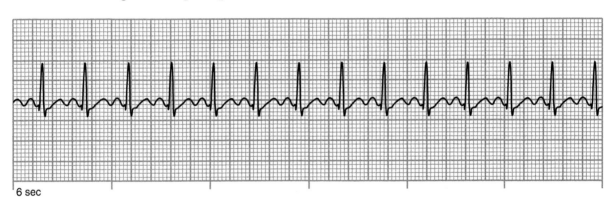

6 sec

6. Rate: between 101 and 150 bpm _____
7. Rhythm regular _____
8. PR: P wave is uniform before each QRS with constant PR intervals _____
9. QRS: uniform (0.04 to 0.11 seconds) _____
10. PR: measurable within normal limits _____

What IS Sinus Bradycardia?

A *sinus bradycardia* occurs when the SA node fires at a rate of less than 60 times per minute and each impulse is conducted through the normal conduction pathway, followed by contraction. Sinus bradycardia, therefore, follows all the same criteria of the NSR, except for the rate, which is less than 60 bpm.

6 sec

Redrawn from Cohn, Gilroy-Doohan: *Flip and see ECG,* Philadelphia, 1996, Saunders, p. 75.

What You NEED TO KNOW

Parasympathetic stimulation or vagal dominance over the SA node most commonly causes sinus bradycardia. The PNS is responsible for the "rest and digest" response. During rest, the PNS, through the vagus nerve, causes the heart rate to slow down. Vagus nerve stimulation can occur when bearing down (**Valsalva maneuver**), such as in defecation or as a result of coughing, vomiting, suctioning, gagging, or carotid sinus massage. An injured SA node, caused by infarction or ischemia (in or surrounding the node) may also cause sinus bradycardia. A sinus bradycardia is often found as a side effect in patient's receiving cardiac medications such as a-blockers.

Sinus bradycardia can be "normal" in athletes who exercise regularly. The heart chambers increase their capacities as the heart muscle thickens (**hypertrophies**) to maintain an adequate cardiac output, despite the lower heart rate.

However, a significant sinus bradycardia will cause cardiac output to be insufficient, and, therefore, cerebral and coronary blood flow will be compromised. This can result in decreased cerebral perfusion, leading to fainting (**Stokes-Adams syndrome**). It can also lead to decreased coronary perfusion, leading to chest pain (**angina**).

Sinus bradycardia is treated only if the patient develops signs of decreased perfusion (e.g., hypotension, decreased level of consciousness, chest pain, shortness of breath). If the patient is stable, as in the case of the patient with an athletic heart, no treatment is necessary.

An antidysrhythmic medication (atropine) is the first-line drug for the treatment of a symptomatic bradycardia. Atropine is classified as a vagolytic, which blocks the influence of the vagus (10th cranial) nerve (vagal effects) on the SA node, thereby allowing the heart rate to increase. If drug therapy fails, a temporary or permanent pacemaker may be necessary. (Pacemakers are also used in conjunction with drug therapy.) Drugs that stimulate the SNS (e.g., dopamine, epinephrine, isoproterenol) may also be used.

If sinus bradycardia occurs because of frequent constipation, stool softeners (docusate sodium) are prescribed to reduce straining during bowel movements. In addition, the health care provider may need to offer nutritional information about fiber and fluid intake.

 Sinus bradycardia may indicate the onset of a sinus arrest; therefore, its presence should always be investigated and a cause determined.

If treatment is effective, the heart rate will increase to between 60 and 100 bpm, while retaining its NSR pattern.

What You DO

To evaluate patients with sinus dysrhythmia, you should do the following:

- Carefully evaluate an ECG strip to determine that the heart rhythm is otherwise normal (except for the slow rate); document it. Severe sinus bradycardia can cause decreased perfusion to vital tissues, leading to fainting (Stokes-Adams syndrome) or organ damage or both.
- If known bradycardic medications (digoxin) are given, record the rate frequently for comparative purposes.
- Observe the rhythm frequently for the presence of ectopic or abnormal beats that suggest that another pacemaker is firing. If ectopic or abnormal beats are present, or if the patient is symptomatic (dizziness, fainting), contact the primary health care provider immediately.
- Counsel the patient about dietary interventions that will reduce constipation (e.g., drink eight 8-ounce glasses of water per day unless contraindicated; increase dietary fiber). These interventions may reduce straining for bowel movements that may stimulate the vagus nerve, reduce heart rate, and cause fainting, particularly in older adults.

Do You UNDERSTAND?

DIRECTIONS: **Examine the following ECG strip. Specify the heart rate, and using the terms *normal*, *abnormal*, *regular*, and *irregular*, specify the ECG features of sinus bradycardia.**

6 sec

1 sec

1. Rate: Brady   40Bpm   abnormal
2. P waves: normal
3. QRS: normal
4. Rhythm: normal
5. PR interval: normal

DIRECTIONS: **List the four cases in which sinus bradycardia may occur.**

6. _____

_____

_____

_____

What IS Sinus Dysrhythmia?

Sinus dysrhythmia is a specific dysrhythmia of the SA node characterized by a slight irregularity in rhythm associated with respiration. Heart rate speeds up with inspiration and slows down with expiration.

6 sec

1 sec

During inspiration, the thoracic cavity enlarges, allowing more blood to enter the heart. The heart rate increases in an attempt to pump out this increased volume. During expiration, the thoracic cavity returns to normal, and blood flow and heart rate slow.

What You NEED TO KNOW

Sinus dysrhythmia is a normal variant, and not considered a cardiac risk, because the rate and rhythm are sufficient to sustain the regular cardiac output and retain the SA node as the pacemaker. It is more typically seen in adolescents and women during periods of extreme stress or exercise. Toddlers can also experience sinus dysrhythmia because of their breathing patterns.

What You DO

If sinus dysrhythmia is identified, no treatment is indicated.
• Recognize that it is a normal variant.
• Document the ECG-obtained rhythm for future comparisons.

 TAKE HOME POINTS

To determine whether a rhythm is a sinus dysrhythmia, you should observe for the following:
• **Rate:** Between 60 and 100 bpm
• **Rhythm:** Slightly irregular or phasic with respiration; the P-P intervals and R-R intervals may vary by 0.12 seconds or more (between the longest and shortest intervals)
• **P wave:** Uniform in shape and present before each QRS complex
• **QRS:** Complexes look alike; 0.04 to 0.11 seconds apart
• **PR interval:** 0.12 to 0.20 seconds

Do You UNDERSTAND?

DIRECTIONS: **Answer the following exercise.**

1. What do NSR, sinus tachycardia, and sinus bradycardia have in common that is not true of sinus dysrhythmia?

_____

_____

_____

DIRECTIONS: **Review the following rhythm strips and place a check mark on the lines below, indicating the characteristics they reveal:**

2.

Redrawn from Cohn, Gilroy-Doohan: *Flip and see ECG,* Philadelphia, 1996, Saunders, p. 75.

3.

Redrawn from Cohn, Gilroy-Doohan: *Flip and see ECG,* Philadelphia, 1996, Saunders, p. 73.

	2		3	
	Yes	No	Yes	No
a. Rate: 60 to 100 bpm	_____	_____	_____	_____
b. Rhythm: Regular	_____	_____	_____	_____
c. P wave: Uniform	_____	_____	_____	_____
d. P wave: Before QRS	_____	_____	_____	_____
e. PR intervals: Within 0.12 to 0.20 sec	_____	_____	_____	_____

4.

Redrawn from Cohn, Gilroy-Doohan: *Flip and see ECG,* Philadelphia, 1996, Saunders, p. 77.

5.

	4		5	
	Yes	No	Yes	No
a. Rate: 60 to 100 bpm	___	___	___	___
b. Rhythm: Regular	___	___	___	___
c. P wave: Uniform	___	___	___	___
d. P wave: Before QRS	___	___	___	___
e. PR intervals: Within 0.12 to 0.20 sec	___	___	___	___

6. What two characteristics did the four strips have in common?

_____

_____

What IS Sinoatrial Arrest or Block?

An SA arrest or block occurs when one or more heartbeats are dropped within an NSR sequence.

1 sec

6 sec   Sinus arrest

If the SA node fails to fire, it is called a *sinus arrest.* No impulse is generated; therefore, there are no P, QRS, or T waves produced. This creates a pause, or flat line, in the ECG for an unpredictable length of time (until the failed SA node recovers and starts to work again). If the pause is too long, a backup pacemaker may generate an escape beat (i.e., a beat or impulse from another site, such as the AV node, atrium, or ventricle, which is generated to prevent compromise to the body from the slowed heart rate). This is a serious condition, as the SA node may fail completely.

If the sinus node fires, but the impulse is blocked from exiting the SA nodal tissue, it is called a *sinus block.* The impulse is generated, but not conducted. This may occur for one or more beats; however, the pause is of a predictable length. Because the SA node continues to fire at its regular rate, the pause lasts exactly the same time interval as the previously conducted beats. P waves can be plotted through the pause. It is this characteristic that differentiates the sinus block from the sinus arrest.

TAKE HOME POINTS
- Both sinus block and sinus arrest result in depolarization failure of atria and ventricles.
- The loss of the P, QRS, and T waveforms creates a pause or flat line on the ECG.
- Sinus blocks and arrests are treated in the same manner.

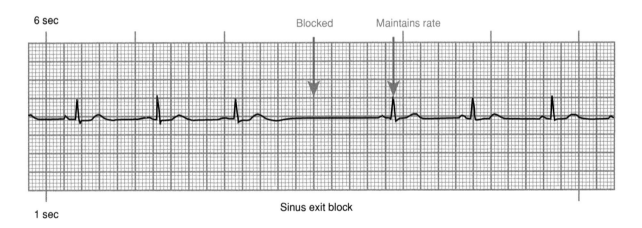

Sinus exit block

What You NEED TO KNOW

In patients with sinoatrial arrest or block, you should remember:
- Treatment is aimed at removing the underlying cause.
- Using calipers or some other reliable form of measurement, you should note whether the next regular beat after the pause maintains the usual P-P and R-R intervals (**cycle length**) in the NSR pattern.
- The usual cause of this sinus dysrhythmia is excessive vagal stimulation of the SA node; this may be evident with overdoses of digitalis glycosides (digoxin), with an antidysrhythmic group IA medication

(quinidine), or with SA node ischemia. (Review the section on *What IS Sinus Bradycardia* for discussion on vagal stimulation.)

- High serum potassium levels (i.e., greater than 5.0 mEq/L), stress, and severe vasoconstriction may also be responsible for sinus dysrhythmia.
- Tight neckwear, heavy lifting, and even hyperextension and rotation of the neck have been known to cause sinus arrest or block.
- If a drug effect is suggested, the drug should be discontinued promptly.
- Heart rhythms need to be carefully monitored whenever new drug therapies are initiated, such as digitalis after a heart attack. In this case, large loading doses of the medication are given and an overdose is possible as reflected in sinus arrest or block.
- The expected outcome of treatment is that the dropped beat or beats will cease or not result in any noticeable change in cardiac output or patient comfort.

If the sinoatrial arrest is prolonged (lasting longer than 3 seconds) or frequent (generally more than 6 per minute, but check hospital policy), an antidysrhythmic (atropine) may be given to inhibit the vagal effect on the SA node. Pacemaker therapy may be needed if other therapy fails.

Heart monitor rate limitations are typically set at 60 for the lower limit and at 100 at the upper limit so that sudden rate changes will trigger the monitor's alarm to sound.

Missed beats may occur frequently or sequentially enough to cause the patient to experience the signs and symptoms of a significant bradycardia and its sequelae. If this occurs, atropine or a permanent pacemaker may be necessary.

!
- Heart rhythms need to be carefully monitored whenever new drug therapies are initiated, such as digitalis after a heart attack.
- Never turn off heart monitor alarms, and be sure to check individual hospital policies for the acceptable monitor limits.

TAKE HOME POINTS

To determine whether a rhythm is SA arrest or block, you should observe the following:
- **Rate:** Usually normal but may be in bradycardic range
- **Rhythm:** *Regular* except for missing beats
- **P wave:** Present and uniform except during the missing beats
- **QRS:** Normal except for the missed beats

What You DO

When SA arrest or block is noted, you should do the following:
- Document the rhythm.
- Differentiate between sinus arrest and sinus block.
- Modify such things as tight neckwear or head hyperextension or rotation to avoid sinus arrest instances (if these are the causes).
- Notify the primary health care provider if it occurs with any regularity or two consecutive beats are missed.
- Notify the health care provider if SA block occurs in relation to giving cardiac medications.

Do You UNDERSTAND?

DIRECTIONS: Indicate in the spaces provided whether the following statements related to sinus block or arrest are *true* or *false*. Suggest a correction for *false* statements.

1. _____ Rate is usually normal but frequently in a bradycardic range.

   _____

   _____

2. _____ P wave is present, but there is no QRS complex.

   _____

   _____

3. _____ There is no QRS complex for the missed beat.

   _____

   _____

DIRECTIONS: Fill in the blanks.

4. Sinus arrest or block can be caused by _____,

   _____, or _____ of the SA

   node.

References

Cummings RO: *ACLS provider manual,* Dallas, 2002, American Heart Association.

Dubin D: *Rapid interpretation of EKGs,* ed 5, Tampa, 1996, Cover Publishing.

Huff J: *ECG workout: exercises in arrhythmia interpretation,* ed 3, Philidelphia, 1997, Lippincott.

Jacobson C: Advanced ECG concepts. In Chulay M, Gizzetta C, Dossey B, editors: *AACN handbook of critical care nursing,* Stamford, Conn, 1998, Appleton & Lange.

Urden LD, Lough ME, Stacy KM: *Thelan's critical care nursing: diagnosis and management,* ed 4, St Louis, 2002, Mosby.

Answers: **1.** true; **2.** false (**P wave is absent**); **3.** true; **4.** excessive vagal stimulation, overdoses of drugs (digitalis, quinidine), ischemia.

NCLEX® Review

1. When reviewing the characteristics of normal sinus rhythm, the health care provider knows that if the sinoatrial node is the dominant pacemaker in a rhythm strip being evaluated, the strip will show:
   1 R-R intervals equal to the PR intervals
   2 A regular rhythm
   3 P waves, consistently rounded and uniform in shape, preceding all QRS complexes
   4 That the dominant pacemaker cannot be determined from a rhythm strip

2. Mr. Peters arrives in the emergency department complaining of palpitations, shortness of breath, and dizziness. His ECG reveals sinus tachycardia. What is the probable cause of his dizziness?
   1 An overstimulation of the parasympathetic nervous system
   2 An increase in cardiac output
   3 A decrease in ventricular filling time
   4 An increase in blood pressure

3. Ms. Houser is a patient with cardiac disease who is now experiencing sinus tachycardia. The health care practitioner is aware that this dysrhythmia could trigger congestive heart failure because:
   1 The cardiac muscle may be unable to sustain the heart rate.
   2 It is well known that this condition occurs with sinus node abnormalities.
   3 The slow heart rate is insufficient to deliver blood to the heart muscle.
   4 Cardiac medications eventually become ineffective, and any dysrhythmia results in heart failure.

4. The heart monitor alarm frequently rings because the patient's usual heart rate of 58 is lower than the preset 60 as lower limit rate. What action should the health care provider take?

1 Turn off the alarm, but look more frequently at the remote ECG screen in the provider's station.
2 Check the hospital's policy, and reset the lower limit to a lower value accordingly.
3 Turn down the alarm, and turn off the graphing device that triggers when the alarm sounds, because monitors are permanently set with their upper and lower limits.
4 Lower the limit on the monitor as necessary because this would be considered an independent-provider judgment.

NCLEX® Review Answers

1. 3 A P wave denotes the conduction of the sinoatrial node stimulus through the atria. The R-R intervals are not equal to PR intervals. Equal R-R intervals define a regular rhythm, but this can be true in nonsinoatrial node–initiated situations, such as nodal tachycardia or ventricular tachycardia. The purpose of evaluating the rhythm strip is to determine information about all aspects of the conduction system, including the dominant pacemaker.

2. 3 Because of the fast heart rate, there is less time for the ventricles to receive full stroke volume. This results in smaller blood volumes with each heartbeat and, therefore, insufficient oxygenation to the brain, resulting in dizziness. Overstimulation of the parasympathetic nervous system would be responsible for an increased heart rate. Although a decrease in cardiac output could account for decreased cerebral perfusion and, thus, dizziness, this is not true of an increase. A decrease rather than an increase in blood pressure might result in insufficient oxygenation to the brain in this particular situation.

3. 1 The increased workload of the heart muscle based on the rapid heart rate can result in decompensation of the muscle, resulting in heart failure. Sinus node abnormalities are not directly known to result in heart failure. Congestive heart failure can occur with any long-term disease related to heart muscle, valvular problems, or high blood pressure. Sinus tachycardia is a rapid heart rate (> 100 bpm), whereas sinus bradycardia is a slow heart rate (< 60 bpm). There is no direct relationship between long-term use of medications and heart failure.

4. 2 Although monitors are typically preset for bradycardia and tachycardia values (< 60 bpm and > 100 bpm), patients are often monitored for these types of dysrhythmias as their underlying cardiac problems. The hospital policy will identify the health care provider's action. The alarm must remain on at all times. Even the most astute provider cannot be expected to observe multiple heart monitors for potentially lethal dysrhythmias. Limits may be changed in accordance with the hospital's policy; other interventions to control the sound or graphing would be inappropriate. The appropriate judgment for the health care provider is that the policy needs to be checked because a constantly sounding alarm defeats the purpose for which it was intended; however, changing it without this review or determination could result in harm to the patient.

Notes

Chapter 9
Practice Strips

Please analyze and identify information for each of the following ECG strips.

Strip 1 Rate: _140 BPM_ ____ Rhythm: _Regular_ ____ P wave: _0.08_ ____

PR interval: _0.12_ ____ QRS: _0.08_ ____

Rhythm interpretation: _Sinus tachycardia_ ____

Strip 2 Rate: _80 Bpm_ ____ Rhythm: _Regular_ ____ P wave: _0.08_ ____

PR interval: _0.12_ ____ QRS: _0.12_ ____

Rhythm interpretation: _Sinus Rythm_ ____

Strip 4   Rate: _80 Bpm_   Rhythm: _normal_   P wave: _0.12_

PR interval: _0.16_   QRS: _0.08_

Rhythm interpretation: _NSR_

Strip 5   Rate: _90 Bpm_   Rhythm: _irregular_   P wave: _neg_

PR interval: _0.04_   QRS: _0.16_

Rhythm interpretation: _NSR_

Strip 6   Rate: _120 Bpm_   Rhythm: _irregular_   P wave: _0.04_

PR interval: _____   QRS: _____

Rhythm interpretation: _____

10 Atrial Dysrhythmias

What You WILL LEARN

After reading this chapter, you will know how to do the following:

✔ Define premature atrial contraction.
✔ Define wandering atrial pacemaker.
✔ Describe supraventricular tachycardia (SVT).
✔ Describe paroxysmal atrial tachycardia.
✔ Define AV nodal reentrant tachycardia (AVNRT).
✔ Differentiate atrial flutter from atrial fibrillation.

The dominant pacemaker of the heart is the sinoatrial (SA) node, because it normally discharges impulses at a rate and rhythm most compatible with human needs. In the heart there are many groups of cells (sites) other than the SA node that have the ability to perform as a pacemaker. These sites, called automaticity foci, act as backup or escape pacemakers if the SA node were to fail. (See "Automaticity" in Chapter 1.)

One mechanism of atrial dysrhythmia occurs when a pacemaker site (**automaticity focus**) in the atria fires before the SA node, not as backup or escape pacemaker, but rather taking over as pacemaker because of irritability, overriding the SA node, either intermittently or continuously. Irritability can be caused by ischemia, electrolyte imbalance, drug toxicity, or hypoxia. Because this irritable focus (pacemaker) is firing abnormally, it is called an **ectopic focus** or an **ectopic pacemaker**. Ectopy or ectopic means outside the normal place and is used to describe any beat originating outside the SA node that is not functioning as a backup pacemaker. Ectopy is usually caused by irritability.

Another mechanism of atrial dysrhythmia is reentry. **Reentry** is the repetitive excitation of a circuit within the conduction pathway. Reentry occurs when an impulse is blocked in one arm (unidirectional) of a small circuit division of the conduction pathway, but travels normally through the rest of the pathway. The impulse traveling normally along the other arm can loop around the blocked area and reenter the circuit, stimulating another impulse.

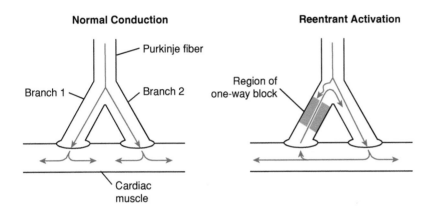

When a pacemaker other than the SA node fires, the P waveforms produced will be different in shape (**morphology**) than the normal waves of SA node. If the ectopic focus is at the top of the atria, the P wave will be upright but shaped differently. If the ectopic focus is near or below the AV node, the P wave may be negative or absent (see illustration on p. 150).

Ectopic foci primarily result from irritability of atrial tissue that is most often caused by increased stimulation of the sympathetic nervous system (SNS) (adrenergic stimulation).

Conditions such as stress and hyperthyroidism increase SNS stimulation by initiating the fight-or-flight response, causing the release of natural adrenergic substances (e.g., epinephrine, norepinephrine). Caffeine, amphetamines, cocaine, alcohol, or other SNS stimulants are also frequently implicated. Lack of oxygen (**hypoxia**) to atrial tissue, electrolyte imbalances (especially hypokalemia), hypothermia, and digitalis toxicity also cause atrial irritability.

Once identified, atrial dysrhythmias are usually treated promptly to preserve cardiac function and control rate. In this chapter, we discuss atrial dysrhythmias in detail to learn about their characteristics, causes, treatments, expected outcomes, and complications.

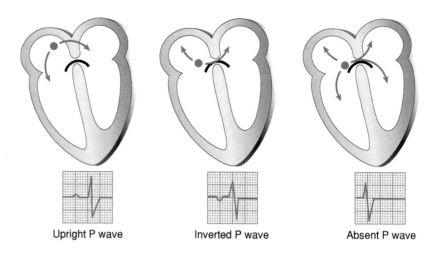

Upright P wave   Inverted P wave   Absent P wave

What IS a Premature Atrial Contraction?

A *premature atrial contraction* (PAC) occurs when an ectopic focus in the atria fires before the next SA node impulse is due. This premature impulse causes atrial depolarization, producing an abnormally shaped P wave on the electrocardiogram (ECG), followed by atrial contraction.

This impulse is conducted to the atrioventricular (AV) node and then to the ventricles, followed by ventricular contraction. The contraction is called *premature* because it happens *before* the next expected heartbeat initiated by the SA node. A slight *noncompensatory pause* occurs after the PAC, before the next normal beat. This pause permits baroreceptors to adjust and the SA node to "reset," reestablishing its rhythm. In this case the next normal beat occurs before expected.

Normal   PAC   Pause

PAC

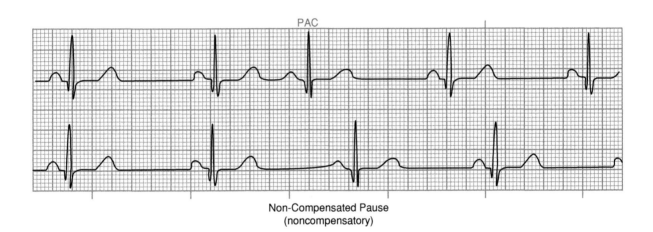

Non-Compensated Pause
(noncompensatory)

PAC   Compensatory Pause

Compensated Pause
(compensatory)

What You NEED TO KNOW

PACs are quite common. Most patients are generally unaware of the PAC and do not experience symptoms. Occasionally, the patient may complain of palpitations or skipped beats. The cause is irritability of the atrial tissue. This irritability may be caused by SNS stimulation, as in anxiety, hypoxia, or ischemia.

Although conducted PACs are most common, some can be nonconducted or aberrantly conducted, producing different waveforms. *Nonconducted PACs* are premature beats that result in only atrial depolarization. This occurs when the AV node from the previous beat does not have time to repolarize before the next impulse arrives. This means that the impulse arrives when the AV node is in the refractory period of repolarization, during which time it cannot be stimulated. Remember, cardiac cells must repolarize for the next depolarization to occur. In this case, the premature impulse is not conducted to the ventricles; therefore neither a QRS complex nor the T wave is recorded on the ECG, and no ventricular contraction occurs.

Unconducted P wave

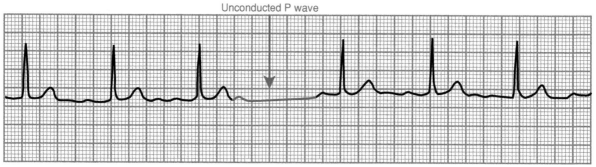

Redrawn from Alpert: *Cardiac arrhythmias,* St Louis, 1980, Mosby, p. 41.

Aberrantly conducted PACs occur when only one of the ventricles from the previous beat has time to repolarize—the other ventricle does not. In this case, one ventricle depolarizes immediately in response to the premature impulse, and the response of the other ventricle is delayed until its repolarization is complete. Aberrantly conducted PACs produce a widened QRS complex on ECG because the ventricles repolarize separately.

Redrawn from Alpert: *Cardiac arrhythmias,* St Louis, 1980, Mosby, p. 36.

When a PAC occurs every other beat (after each normal beat), it is called *atrial bigeminy.* When a PAC occurs every third beat (after every two normal beats), it is called *atrial trigeminy.*

Atrial bigeminy

Redrawn from Alpert: *Cardiac arrhythmias,* St Louis, 1980, Mosby, p. 39.

Atrial trigeminy

Drugs such as caffeine, nicotine, amphetamines, marijuana, catecholamines, and anesthetic agents or diseases (hyperthyroidism) may enhance PACs.

If PACs occur infrequently and do not increase to more than six per minute, treatment is usually unnecessary. However, if PACs occur with increased frequency, antidysrhythmic group IA drugs (e.g., quinidine) may be given.

The expected outcome of treatment is that the PACs will cause no changes in cardiac output or patient comfort and will not increase to more than six per minute. Increased frequency of PACs may lead to more serious dysrhythmias, such as atrial fibrillation.

Watch for the development of more serious atrial dysrhythmias such as atrial tachycardia, flutter, or fibrillation. These indicate more serious atrial irritability.

What You DO

- Identify and document the rhythm.
- Distinguish PACs from other forms of irregular rhythms; that is, look for P waves, check their shapes, and determine whether they are followed by QRS complexes and noncompensatory pauses.
- Document PACs via ECG strips.
- Count the number of PACs occurring per minute, and notify the health care provider if there are more than six per minute or a progressive increase from the occasional PAC. Treatment is usually not required unless the patient is symptomatic.
- Once identified, teach the patient about lifestyle changes that can and should be used, such as stress reduction, limiting caffeine and alcohol intake, and adequate rest with exercise.

TAKE HOME POINTS

To determine whether a rhythm includes a PAC, you should observe for the following:

- **Rate:** Usually unaffected
- **Rhythm:** Normal except for the premature beat and noncompensatory pause
- **P wave:** Either abnormally shaped or inverted; will be different in shape (i.e., morphology) from sinus node P waves; may also be buried in T wave of the preceding beat
- **PR interval:** Can be shortened or prolonged but will be different from the PR intervals of SA node
- **QRS:** Usually unaffected (i.e., 0.04 to 0.11) and follows the P wave; may be aberrantly conducted (> 0.11) or nonconducted

Do You UNDERSTAND?

DIRECTIONS: **Fill in the blanks.**

1. A beat is called _premature atrial contraction_ when some ectopic pacemaker fires ahead of the SA node.
2. A contraction called a PAC occurs when the _atrial_ tissue is irritable.
3. In most instances, a _QRS_ follows a P wave in the PAC.

DIRECTIONS: **Complete the following exercises.**

4. Which of the numbered complexes in the following ECG strip are PACs?
   _2, 4, 9_

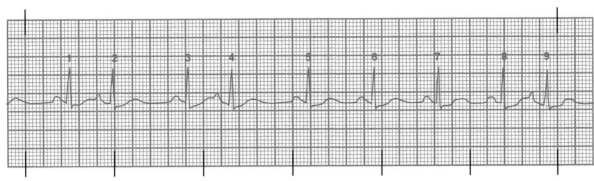

Redrawn from Cohn, *Gilroy-Doohan: Flip and see ECG,* Philadelphia, 1996, Saunders, p. 79.

5. Compare the T waves preceding QRS complexes three and four.
   Why are they different?

   _____

   _____

DIRECTIONS: **Fill in the blanks.**

6. The larger space between complex four and five is called the
   _____ _____ and occurs

   because _____.

What IS a Wandering Atrial Pacemaker?

A *wandering atrial pacemaker* (WAP) occurs when the pacemaker site shifts or *wanders* from the SA node to different pacemaker sites in the atria and back again. The morphology of the P wave changes according to the pacemaker site where the impulse has originated. It is caused by increased parasympathetic (vagal) stimulation that causes the SA node to slow down, allowing another pacemaker to take over. There are usually at least three different foci firing in the atria, so there will be at least three different shapes of P waves on the ECG. The firing rate will vary slightly, but it usually remains between 60 and 100 beats per minute (bpm). If the

LIFE SPAN

WAP is not considered serious; it is found in the very young, frequently in athletes.

Answers: 5. The T wave for QRS complex four contains the P wave of the PAC and therefore looks larger or is shaped differently from the other T waves 6. noncompensatory pause, the SA node is reset to reestablish the ventricular rate.

rate increases to greater than 100 bpm, the dysrhythmia is called *multi-focal atrial tachycardia* (MAT). MAT is seen in patients with chronic obstructive pulmonary disease (COPD) or serious heart disease. It is essentially the same as WAP; however, the rate is greater than 100 bpm.

Redrawn from Phipps, Sands, Marek: *Medical-surgical nursing: concepts and clinical practice,* ed 6, St Louis, 1999, Mosby, p. 670.

TAKE HOME POINTS

To determine whether a rhythm is a WAP, observe the following:

- **Rate:** Usually normal (between 60 and 100 bpm); however, it may slow if there is vagal dominance. If greater than 100 bpm, it is a MAT.
- **Rhythm:** Irregular; intervals increase and decrease as the pacemaker shifts between the SA node and other atrial pacemakers.
- **P wave:** Primary characteristic is the differences in the shape of the P waves that reflect different sites of origin.
- **PR interval:** Variable and may be difficult to measure at times.
- **QRS complexes:** Follows all P waves.
- **QT:** Measurable and within normal limits.
- **MAT:** May be called a supraventricular (i.e., above the ventricles) tachycardia, because the rhythm originates from pacemakers in the atria that are above the ventricles.

SA node

What You NEED TO KNOW

There is generally a dominance of vagal stimulation or a drug, such as a digitalis glycoside (e.g., digoxin), to be given to cause WAP. In most cases, the patient experiences no symptoms and no treatment is necessary. However, an antidysrhythmic (e.g., atropine) may be prescribed if the rate slows too much (i.e., less than 60) causing symptoms.

It is expected that the wandering pacemaker will not result in a permanent shift in the dominant pacemaker, and the cardiac output will be sufficiently sustained. If MAT occurs, treatment is directed toward eliminating the irritability and slowing the ventricular rate.

What You DO

- Document the rhythm.
- If a drug (e.g., digitalis) is the suggested cause, you should withhold it, notify the primary care provider and monitor the rhythm.

Do You UNDERSTAND?

DIRECTIONS: **Fill in the blanks.**

1. If the health care provider suspects a WAP, what component of waveform should be evaluated? _____

Redrawn from Paul, Hebra: *The nurse's guide to cardiac rhythm interpretation,* Philadelphia, 1998, Saunders, p. 89.

Answer: 1. **P wave.**

2. The QRS complexes are numbered 1 through 10.
   a. Which complexes are most likely to have been initiated by the atria above the AV node?

   _____

   b. Which complexes are most likely to have been initiated by the atria at or below the AV node? _____

   c. Which complexes are most likely to have been initiated by the ventricle? _____

What IS Supraventricular Tachycardia?

Supraventricular tachycardia (SVT) is a term used to describe any tachycardic rhythm originating in or above the bundle of His (supra—above, ventricular—the ventricles). SVTs can include sinus tachycardia, atrial fibrillation, and atrial flutter. An SVT may be described as **paroxysmal** (PSVT) if it begins and/or ends abruptly. The word paroxysmal means sudden onset or sudden cessation. In the clinical setting, however, the term PSVT does not describe all of the supraventricular tachycardias, instead it is reserved for two particular rhythms; **paroxysmal atrial tachycardia** and **atrioventricular (AV) nodal reentrant tachycardia**. Another type of PSVT occurs in patients with accessory conduction pathways and will be discussed in a later chapter.

✱Cessation = Stop

What IS Paroxysmal Atrial Tachycardia? 150-250 BPM

Paroxysmal atrial tachycardia (PAT) is the *sudden* onset of a rapid, ectopic, atrial rhythm. A very irritable ectopic focus in the atria takes over as pacemaker, firing at rates of 150 to 250 bpm. Because the impulse is generated from a different pacemaker than the SA node, the P waves produced are different in shape from the SA node–generated P waves. The impulse travels down the normal conduction pathway, producing normal QRS

Answers: 2a. 2, 5, 6, 7, 8, 9; 2b. 1, 4, 10; 2c. 3.

and T waves followed by contraction. In contrast with sinus tachycardia, in which the SA node gradually increases rate in response to exercise or excitement, PAT begins and ends abruptly. One or more PACs usually precede PAT. PAT can last for minutes, to days.

In patients with no history of cardiac disease, PAT is caused by SNS stimulation as seen with emotional stress and anxiety, excessive caffeine, and alcohol and tobacco use. PAT may also be seen with myocardial infarction and states of hypoxia.

What You NEED TO KNOW

In patients with rapid rates (greater than 200 bpm), hypokalemia, or high blood levels of digitalis, conduction may be blocked, which is called *PAT with block*. PAT with block occurs when the AV node is not able to respond to the rapid number of impulses being sent from the ectopic atrial focus. When this happens, the AV node will selectively conduct only a certain number of impulses down to the ventricles; all others will be blocked. PAT with block is identified when there is a P wave with no QRS or T wave after it, because conduction to the ventricles was blocked at the AV node. Blocks may occur with every other P wave (i.e., a 2:1 ratio of P wave to QRS) or variably.

The rapid rate decreases ventricular filling time, resulting in decreased cardiac output and increased myocardial oxygen consumption. Treatment goals for PAT are aimed at reducing the ventricular rate and decreasing the cause of irritability.

The young may tolerate PAT because of their normal fast heart rate and their ability to compensate; however, it may make older patients feel light-headed and fatigued.

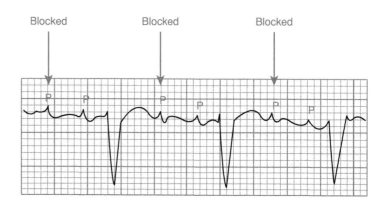

Blocked   Blocked   Blocked

> • Carotid massage is another form of vagal maneuver, but it should not be performed by nurses.
> • A life-threatening dysrhythmia may occur if the shock is delivered at the peak or downward slope of the T wave. Cardioversion is used if the patient is unstable or if drug therapy failed.

TAKE HOME POINTS

To determine whether the rhythm is PAT, you should observe for the following:
- **Rate:** *Atrial:* 150 to 250 bpm; *Ventricular:* Varies, depending on whether there is any degree of AV block
- **Rhythm:** Regular, unless there is a variable block
- **P wave:** Different in morphology to the SA node–generated P wave (May be hidden in the T wave of the preceding beat.)
- **PR interval:** Difficult to measure
- **QRS:** Normal 0.04 to 0.11 (Conduction beyond the AV node is normal; QRS may be absent if the conduction is blocked, and it may be wide if aberrantly conducted.)

What You DO

- Identify and document the rhythm. Note whether PAT is occurring with block.
- Monitor for signs of hypoperfusion and myocardial ischemia, such as syncope, hypotension, and chest pain.
- For stable patients, maneuvers to stimulate the vagus nerve (vagal maneuvers) of the parasympathetic nervous system (PNS), such as bearing down or tightening abdominal muscles (**Valsalva maneuver**) or carotid massage, are used. Vagal maneuvers suppress automaticity and decrease conduction through the AV node, resulting in a slower heart rate.
- If vagal maneuvers fail, drug therapy with an antidysrhythmic (adenosine) can be initiated. Adenosine is the drug of choice for PAT; however, digoxin may be used to slow the ventricular rate and convert the rhythm-to-sinus rhythm, but it must be used with caution because it may cause PAT with block. β-blockers or calcium channel blockers may also be used to slow the ventricular rate and convert the rhythm. Quinidine may be added to prevent the recurrence of PAT.
- For the unstable patient (i.e., the patient exhibiting syncope, hypotension, or chest pain), cardioversion will be necessary.

  Cardioversion is similar to defibrillation, but less wattage may be used (i.e., 50 to 360 J), and it is not considered an emergency procedure. The patient is premedicated with a sedative (usually diazepam), but is conscious (the shock may be momentarily painful). The shock is synchronized with the R wave of the ECG pattern to avoid precipitating ventricular fibrillation.

Do You UNDERSTAND?

DIRECTIONS: **Fill in the blanks.**
1. Paroxysmal means _____.
2. In PAT, the atrial rate ranges from 150 to _____ bpm.
3. PAT with block occurs in patients with high blood levels of
   _____.
4. Aberrant conduction through the ventricles will produce a QRS
   complex that is _____.
5. PAT can be seen in patients with _____
   cardiac history.

What IS AV Nodal Reentrant Tachycardia?

AV nodal reentrant tachycardia (AVNRT) is a reentrant tachycardia caused by a reentry circuit in or near the AV node. It is usually triggered by a PAC, resulting in rates of 150 to 250 beats per minute. It is a regular rhythm, typically with a narrow QRS complex. The P waves are usually hidden within the preceding T wave due to the rapid rate.

What You NEED TO KNOW

AVNRT is the most common type of PSVT. It is usually well tolerated in patients with no structural heart disease. It may cause myocardial infarction in patients with coronary artery disease (CAD). It is more common in young adults and seen more often in women than in men. Syncope may occur due to decreased ventricular filling time causing decreased cardiac output, hypotension, and reduced cerebral circulation.

What You DO

- Identify and document the rhythm. Begin supplemental oxygen.
- Monitor for signs of hypoperfusion and myocardial ischemia, such as syncope, hypotension, and chest pain.
- For stable patients, vagal maneuvers (see earlier) are recommended.
- Drug therapy should be initiated if vagal maneuvers fail. Intravenous drug therapy includes adenosine, short-acting calcium channel blockers, or β-blockers, or amiodarone.
- For the patient with prolonged tachycardia, synchronized cardioversion (see earlier) will be necessary to prevent shock.
- Radiofrequency catheter ablation (RFCA) of the reentrant circuit is considered for the patient with frequent, recurrent episodes or the patient who fails drug therapy.

Do You UNDERSTAND?

DIRECTIONS: **Fill in the blanks.**
1. The most common type of PSVT is _____.
2. AVNRT is usually triggered by a _____.
3. Initial therapy for AVNRT should include _____.
4. The rhythm seen in AVNRT is _____.

TAKE HOME POINTS

To determine whether the rhythm is AVNRT, you should observe for the following:
- **Rate:** *Ventricular:* 150 to 250 beats/min; more common in the 180 to 200 beats/min range
- **Rhythm:** Regular
- **P wave:** Usually hidden in the T wave of the preceding beat.
- **PR interval:** Unable to measure
- **QRS:** Normal 0.04 to 0.10 QRS may be wide if there is an intraventricular conduction delay.

What IS Atrial Flutter? 250-350 BPm

In *atrial flutter,* atrial depolarization occurs at rates of 250 to 350 times per minute, resulting in ineffective atrial contractions, with a variable

Answers: 1. AVNRT; 2. PAC; 3. vagal maneuvers; 4. regular.

ventricular response of 60 to 150 bpm. Between ventricular contractions or the QRS complex, the atrial activity is seen as *sawtoothed* or flutter waves. The mechanism behind this dysrhythmia is believed to be "reentry." In this mechanism, a pacing impulse loops around a fixed obstacle within a defined circuit and reenters the circuit rapidly, initiating another impulse. The AV node is not able to respond to the large number of impulses; therefore it selectively conducts only a certain number of impulses down to the ventricles; all others are blocked.

Depending on the number of sawtoothed waves between ventricular contractions, the rhythm is referred to as atrial flutter with 2:1, 3:1, or 4:1 block. If the ventricular block rate or *conduction ratio* remains the same (**fixed**), the rhythm will then be regular. If the ventricular block rate or conduction ratio varies, the rhythm will be irregular.

What You NEED TO KNOW

The presence of atrial flutter can only be documented via ECG and not by listening to or counting the pulse (even an apical pulse). The rhythm of the pulse can be regular or irregular. If there is a high degree of block (e.g., an atrial rate of 300 with a 4:1 block that yields a ventricular rate of 75), the effect on the ventricle may be minimal.

Atrial flutter can occur alone, but it tends to occur in association with COPD, high blood pressure, heart muscle abnormalities, heart failure, coronary artery disease, and hyperthyroidism. Atrial flutter can be treated pharmacologically or by cardioversion (see the discussion of cardioversion earlier in the chapter).

Pharmacologic therapy involves the use of digitalis glycosides (e.g., digoxin), β-adrenergic blockers (e.g., metoprolol), or calcium

⚠ Rapid ventricular rates result in decreased ventricular filling time, which diminishes cardiac output and increases myocardial oxygen consumption. This decrease in cardiac output with increased workload can result in chest pain or left ventricular heart failure if the condition remains untreated. If the patient exhibits these symptoms of instability, synchronized cardioversion is recommended.

Once the ventricular rate is under control, an antidysrhythmic (e.g., quinidine, amiodarone) may be added to convert the rhythm. If treatment is effective, it is expected that the patient will return to normal sinus rhythm (NSR) with sufficient cardiac output.

⚠ Observe the cardiac monitor carefully. Depending on the degree of block, the high-rate alarm may or may not sound.

channel blockers (e.g., diltiazem) to slow the ventricular response. Anticoagulant therapy may be recommended, as blood in the atria may pool secondary to ineffective contractions resulting in clot formations.

If the ventricular response is rapid, the patient may complain of palpitations, angina, or dizziness. With rapid ventricular rates, cardiac output is diminished, and myocardial oxygen consumption is increased. Atrial flutter with a ventricular rate greater than 100 bpm may be called a *supraventricular tachycardia,* because the rhythm originates from a pacemaker in the atrium that is above the ventricles.

What You DO

- Identify the dysrhythmia, document via ECG strip, and notify the health care provider.
- Determine whether the patient is symptomatic (i.e., the patient has chest pain or dizziness), and assess vital signs.
- If drugs are used, monitor rhythm for effectiveness in converting or sustaining NSR.
- Assist with cardioversion as necessary.

Do You UNDERSTAND?

DIRECTIONS: **Complete the following exercises.**
1. Specify the ventricular rate for each of the following situations.
    a. Atrial rate of 300 with 3:1 block = _____
    b. Atrial rate of 240 with 4:1 block = _____
    c. Atrial rate of 250 with 2:1 block = _____
    d. Atrial rate of 150 with 1:1 block = _____

Answers: **1a.** 100; **1b.** 60; **1c.** 125; **1d.** 150.

**DIRECTIONS: Atrial flutter can occur with varying degrees of ventric-
ular block. Examine the following ECG strip, and fill in
the blanks.**

Redrawn from Paul, Hebra: *The nurse's guide to cardiac rhythm interpretation,* Philadelphia, 1998, Saunders, p. 100.

2. a. What is the atrial rate for 1 minute? _____
   b. What is the ventricular rate for 1 minute? _____

What IS Atrial Fibrillation? 400 + Bpm

In *atrial fibrillation,* there are multiple reentry circuits in the atria, resulting in chaotic impulse formation and producing impulses at rates of 400
or more per minute. The atria are not able to recover before an additional
impulse fires again; thus neither atria ever fully depolarizes. The result is
quivering or fibrillation of the atria instead of contraction. Because the
atria never fully depolarize, no discernable P waves are produced. Only
a series of tiny, erratic spikes are produced. Sometimes the spikes are so
tiny that they appear to be a wavy baseline.

SA node

The AV node is not able to respond to the large number of impulses from the multiple reentry circuits; it conducts impulses in a totally unpredictable or erratic manner, resulting in an irregular ventricular response. The heart rhythm in atrial fibrillation is called *irregularly irregular*, which means that not only is the rhythm irregular, but it also has no predictable pattern. Occasionally, the ventricles may respond aberrantly. (See the discussion of aberrantly conducted PAC.)

Treatment goals for atrial fibrillation are to eliminate or decrease the cause of the atrial irritability and to decrease the ventricular rate.

What You NEED TO KNOW

The patient is generally aware of atrial fibrillation when the heart rate is uncontrolled and palpitations may be experienced. In atrial fibrillation, the patient's pulse remains irregular whenever it is palpated, auscultated, or measured. Ventricular rates should be assessed using the *6-second method* (see Chapter 4). If the rate is less than 100 bpm, the rhythm is called atrial fibrillation with a controlled ventricular response or *controlled atrial fibrillation*.

If the rate is greater than 100 bpm, the rhythm is called atrial fibrillation with a rapid ventricular response (RVR) or *uncontrolled atrial fibrillation*.

Normal atrial contraction provides 25% to 30% of cardiac output. Atrial contraction is clinically called *atrial kick*. In atrial fibrillation, atrial contraction or atrial kick is lost. As such, the atria do not completely empty its contents into the ventricles. This results in blood pooling in the atria and decreased cardiac output. The treatment for atrial fibrillation is dependent on the rate of ventricular response and the degree of circulatory insufficiency the patient experiences.

If the patient is unstable (i.e., experiencing chest pain or heart failure) or if drug therapy fails, cardioversion to restore the SA node as pacemaker may be attempted.

Drug therapy includes the following:
- Amiodarone, an antidysrhythmic agent
- Digitalis glycoside (digoxin). It increases the refractory or resting time of the AV node, resulting in a controlled ventricular response that the patient can then tolerate.
- β-adrenergic blockers (metoprolol)
- Calcium channel blockers (diltiazem) slow the ventricular response. An antidysrhythmic (quinidine, amiodarone) may decrease atrial irritability.

Treatment for controlled atrial fibrillation of long-standing origin may be solely directed toward eliminating the cause of the atrial irritability. As a result of treatment, it is expected that the patient will sustain a controlled ventricular response with adequate evidence of sufficient overall circulation.

- Atrial fibrillation with a rapid ventricular response is considered very serious.
- The major threat, particularly in the instance of a heart attack, is inadequacy of cardiac output. This output is decreased approximately 25% when atrial contraction is not contributing to ventricular filling.

The formation of small blood clots that accumulate on the walls of the atria as a result of pooling is a major threat. In addition to this problem, the blood is also agitated by the fibrillation, which accelerates normal clotting. Thrombi can become emboli, resulting in pulmonary emboli, heart attack, or stroke, depending on their final resting place. Anticoagulants may be prescribed.

The major threat, particularly in the instance of a heart attack, is inadequacy of cardiac output. This output is decreased approximately 25% when atrial contraction is not contributing to ventricular filling. Therefore heart failure and further ischemia are of grave concern.

Another major threat is the formation of small blood clots (**mural thrombi**) that accumulate on the walls of the atria as a result of pooling. In addition to the problem with pooling, the blood is also agitated by the fibrillation, which accelerates normal clotting. Thrombi can become emboli, resulting in pulmonary emboli, heart attack, or stroke, depending on their final resting place. Anticoagulants (e.g., heparin sulfate, warfarin sodium) may be prescribed to reduce the threat of clot formation, particularly around heart valves in long-standing atrial fibrillation.

Atrial fibrillation with a rapid ventricular response may be called a supraventricular tachycardia, because the rhythm originates from pacemakers in the atria that are above the ventricles.

What You DO

- If atrial fibrillation develops suddenly, document it, notify the physician, and prepare for the possibility of cardioversion, administration of intravenous amiodarone, digitalis glycoside (e.g., digoxin), or both.
- Whether acute or chronic, you should monitor the vital signs for evidence of sufficiency of cardiac output.
- Be alert for any signs that emboli have been released from atria walls, such as sudden onset of chest pain or shortness of breath (heart attack or pulmonary emboli), cool extremities (clots to lower arterial system), or change in level of consciousness or muscle movement (stroke).
- Monitor coagulation studies (heparin = partial thromboplastin time [PTT]; warfarin sodium = prothrombin time [PT]) and the international normalized ratio (INR) if anticoagulants are prescribed. Patients with chronic atrial fibrillation who then become bedridden or sedentary for other health problems add the risk for emboli to their health concerns.
- If digitalis glycoside (e.g., digoxin) or antidysrhythmia medication (e.g., amiodarone) is given, monitor the patient for toxicity if the heart

rate suddenly increases or decreases. This monitoring is done through blood-level determinations.

- Monitor the radial or apical pulse. The palpated radial pulse may feel not only irregular in rhythm but also irregular in volume because irregular amounts of blood are being circulated.

Do You UNDERSTAND?

DIRECTIONS: Complete the following exercises.

1. Name three ways that atrial fibrillation differs from atrial flutter.

   _____

   _____

   _____

2. In a patient in NSR, if there is electrical interference on the monitor or the patient is moving, the tracing between QRS complexes can be erratic or nondistinct. What could the health care provider do to test the difference between that interference situation and atrial fibrillation?

   _____

   _____

   _____

   _____

TAKE HOME POINTS

To determine whether a rhythm is atrial fibrillation, you should observe for the following:

- **Rate:** Varies according to ventricular response (< 100 = controlled atrial fibrillation; > 100 = uncontrolled atrial fibrillation; < 100 increases stroke volume for each ventricular contraction, thus improves overall circulation with each heartbeat)
- **Rhythm:** Irregularly irregular
- **P wave:** No true P waves (varying F waves—from course to fine—may be seen)
- **PR interval:** Not measurable
- **QRS:** Usually normal, but may be aberrant

TAKE HOME POINTS

Generally, patients will know if their heart rate is irregular. Immediate concerns of the health care provider can be dispelled by asking this simple question, "Has anyone ever told you that your heartbeat is irregular?"

LIFE SPAN

Atrial flutter and fibrillation may occur more often in the older patient who has a history of hypertension, CAD, and myocardial infarctions. These health problems may damage the conduction system over time, and the arrhythmia may be treated as a chronic problem. Older patients should also be cautioned about sudden postural changes (e.g., quickly moving from a lying to a sitting or standing position). These sudden movements may result in fainting if atrial dysrhythmias have altered cerebral blood supply and perfusion.

Answers: 1. **Atrial rate (400 bpm versus 250 to 350 bpm), degree of AV block (no set pattern versus 1:1, 2:1, 3:1, or 4:1), can be chronic and not treated versus an acute situation that requires cardioversion or drugs; 2. The QRS complexes in atrial fibrillation will be spaced irregularly irregular from each other, those in NSR will be equidistant. The ventricular rate will be relatively constant in NSR, the rate in atrial fibrilla- tion will vary.**

References

American College of Cardiology Foundation, American Heart Association: *ACC/AHA/ESC guidelines for the management of patients with supraventricular arrythmias,* 2004. Available at www.acc.org/clinical/guidelines/arrhythmias/III_general.htm.

Blomstrom-Lundqvist C et al: ACC/AHA/ESC guidelines for the management of patients with supraventricular arrythmias—executive summary, *J Am Coll Cardiol* 42(8):1493-1531, 2003.

Clark A: Atrial flutter, *EMedicine,* 2004. Available at www.emedicine.com?emerg/topic47.htm.

Cummings RO: *ACLS provider manual,* Dallas, 2002, American Heart Association.

Dubin D: *Rapid interpretation of EKGs,* ed 5, Tampa, 1996, Cover Publishing.

Huff J: *ECG workout: exercises in arrhythmia interpretation,* ed 3, Philadelphia, 1997, Lippincott.

Jacobson C: Advanced ECG concepts. In Chulay M, Gizzetta C, Dossey B, editors: *AACN handbook of critical care nursing,* Stamford, Conn, 1998, Appleton & Lange.

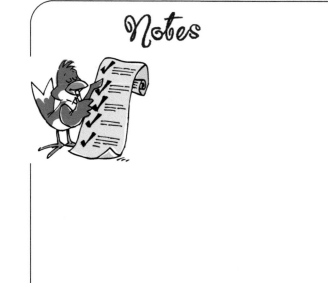

Notes

NCLEX® Review

1. Mr. Willow's ECG shows five premature atrial contractions in a 1-minute strip. What action should the health care practitioner take?
   1 Notify the physician immediately because these ectopic beats may quickly lead to life-threatening dysrhythmias.
   2 Disregard these beats but take the patient's blood pressure more often to access cardiac output.
   3 Change the patient's dietary order to include only decaffeinated beverages.
   4 Monitor Mr. Willow's ECG and notify the physician if six or more premature atrial contractions occur in a 1-minute strip.

2. The health care provider is assessing the patient's apical rate, which is very irregular at a varying rate of 60 to 150 bpm. What might the provider conclude from this assessment?
   1 The patient is in atrial flutter with a varying degree of block.
   2 The patient is in atrial fibrillation because this would be heard as an irregular heartbeat.
   3 The patient's ECG needs to be observed to determine the nature of the dysrhythmia.
   4 The patient is in an accelerated junctional tachycardia because a varying rate is a hallmark feature of this dysrhythmia.

3. Ms. Belfry has been diagnosed with atrial flutter and is scheduled for a cardioversion. When assisting with this procedure, the health care practitioner anticipates that the shock will be given at what point on the ECG waveform?
   1 On the P wave
   2 On the R wave
   3 On the T wave
   4 During the PR interval

4. The health care provider suspects that a patient with a paroxysmal supraventricular tachycardia may be experiencing a decrease in cardiac output. Which of the following assessment findings supports this concern?
   1 Flushed face and warm extremities
   2 Capillary refill less than 3 seconds
   3 A complaint of chest pain, subsiding as output lowers and oxygen demands decrease
   4 Dizziness when the patient sits in a chair

5. The heart conduction system includes inherent pacemakers at varying locations. Which of the following ECG tracing descriptions might the health care provider observe if the atrioventricular node were the primary pacemaker?
   1 Absence of P waves and a ventricular rate less than 40 bpm
   2 Abnormally shaped QRS complexes
   3 Absent or inverted P waves and a ventricular rate between 40 and 60 bpm
   4 Depressed ST segments

6. A patient's heart rate has decreased over several days from 70 to 54 bpm. Which of the following drugs may be responsible for the change?
   1 Adenosine (Adenocard)
   2 Furosemide (Lasix)
   3 Digoxin (Lanoxin)
   4 Atropine (atropine sulfate, Isopto Atropine)

7. Mr. Carson develops paroxysmal supraventricular tachycardia during a time of high stress in his life. Despite efforts to reduce his stress, his condition continues. What initial therapy might be attempted to end paroxysmal supraventricular tachycardia?
   1 Vagal stimulation
   2 Cardioversion
   3 Intravenous adenosine (Adenocard)
   4 Intravenous epinephrine (adrenaline)

NCLEX® Review Answers

1. **4** The new development of six or more premature atrial contractions in 1 minute would be cause for notifying the physician, because their presence suggests a possible new irritability that should be investigated further. Fewer than six premature atrial contractions per minute are not considered life threatening. In general, the health care provider should be aware of new developments in rhythms. Therefore if Mr. Willow developed premature atrial contractions when none were evident before, it would be good to alert the physician on the next regular contact; however, this is not an emergency. Provided there is not a significant change in the ventricular rate of this patient, cardiac output should not be changed. Caffeinated beverages can contribute to premature atrial contractions, but the practitioner would not be the one initiating a dietary change.

2. **3** Although it is possible to use the generic labels of bradycardia or tachycardia for slow and rapid heart rates, respectively, precise dysrhythmias can only be documented with an ECG. It is not possible to identify atrial flutter, atrial fibrillation, or accelerated junctional tachycardia through auscultation.

3. **2** This type of shock is called synchronous cardioversion; a shock at this time directs conduction and systole to occur simultaneously, reestablishing the normal conduction pathway. Once the P wave is initiated, the QRS would follow and the conduction system would not be reset. The T wave is the time for ventricular repolarization or diastole; a shock at this time would be dangerous because the ventricle should not be contracting and life-threatening dysrhythmias can result (ventricular fibrillation).

4. **4** Dizziness occurs because of the reduced stroke volume (a result of shortened ventricular filling time) with the rapid rate and the small subsequent quantities of blood perfusing the cerebral tissue. Warm face and extremities would suggest that cardiac output is adequate. Capillary refill should be less than 3 seconds if there is sufficient cardiac output. Lower oxygen demands on the myocardium decrease chest pain, but this occurs when cardiac output is sufficient and not lowered.

5. **3** Abnormal or inverted P waves and a ventricular rate between 40 and 60 bpm suggests that the atrioventricular node is the primary pacemaker because atrial contraction is seen in retrograde fashion as inverted P waves. The absence of P waves and a ventricular rate less than 40 bpm suggests that the ventricular tissue is the primary pacemaker. Abnormally shaped QRS complexes suggest abnormal conduction in the bundle of His or may refer to QRS complexes seen in premature ventricular contractions. Depressed ST segments suggest myocardial injury. Elevated ST segments suggest myocardial ischemia or oxygen deficiency.

6. **3** Digoxin, as a chronotropic drug, promotes a decrease in rate because it prolongs the refractory (resting) time of the atrioventricular node. Fewer sinoatrial or atrial stimuli are thus conducted to the ventricle and the heart rate decreases. Adenosine is used to suppress paroxysmal supraventricular tachycardia. Furosemide is a loop diuretic; it promotes water elimination and, thus, can assist in the reduction of blood pressure, but it does not directly lower heart rate. Atropine is given to increase heart rate and is used in the treatment of bradycardia.

7. **1** Stimulation of the vagus nerve through carotid massage, eyeball pressure, or initiation of the Valsalva maneuver (bearing down, as in defecation) may be successful in reducing the heart rate and is the initial approach to paroxysmal supraventricular tachycardia in most patients. Cardioversion may be tried when vagal stimulation and drug therapy fail. Adenosine is the drug of choice and is usually given if vagal stimulation is unsuccessful. Epinephrine would increase the heart rate and is not used in paroxysmal supraventricular tachycardia.

Chapter 10
Practice Strips

Please analyze and identify information for each of the following ECG strips.

Strip 1   Rate: _____   Rhythm: _____   P wave: _____

PR interval: _____   QRS: _____

Rhythm interpretation: _____

Strip 2   Rate: _____ Rhythm: _____ P wave: _____

PR interval: _____ QRS: _____

Rhythm interpretation: _____

Strip 3   Rate: _____ Rhythm: _____ P wave: _____

PR interval: _____ QRS: _____

Rhythm interpretation: _____

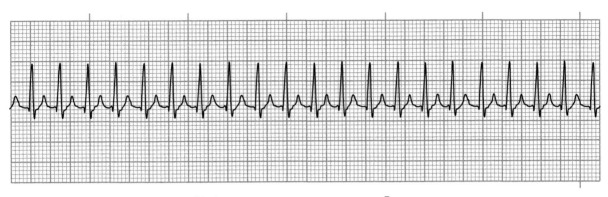

Strip 4   Rate: _____ Rhythm: _____ P wave: _____

PR interval: _____ QRS: _____

Rhythm interpretation: _____

Strip 5   Rate: _____ Rhythm: _____ P wave: _____

PR interval: _____ QRS: _____

Rhythm interpretation: _____

Strip 6   Rate: _____   Rhythm: _____   P wave: _____

PR interval: _____   QRS: _____

Rhythm interpretation: _____

Junctional Dysrhythmias

What You WILL LEARN

After reading this chapter, you will know how to do the following:

- ✔ Define AV junctional (nodal) rhythm.
- ✔ Define premature junctional contraction.
- ✔ Define junctional tachycardia.
- ✔ Describe SVT/PSVT.
- ✔ Describe the rate parameters associated with an accelerated junctional rhythm.

automaticity = initiate

The atrioventricular (AV) node is an area of tissue located on the posterior floor of the right atrium. This tissue is a connector between the atrial and ventricular conduction pathways. The AV junctional tissue includes the AV node and the tissue immediately surrounding it.

Junctional rhythms, which are sometimes referred to as **nodal rhythms**, are the result of two primary causes: (1) failure of the sinoatrial (SA) node to generate an impulse and (2) increased automaticity of the junctional tissue. If the SA node fails to generate an impulse either because of a disease or suppression by drugs, it may cease to serve as the primary pacemaker of the heart, and the AV node will work as a compensatory pacemaker to generate an impulse. Normally when the AV junction acts as a compensatory pacemaker, it has the ability to generate impulses at a rate of 40 to 60 beats per minute (bpm). Rhythms also originate from the AV junctional tissue because of increased automaticity of this tissue resulting from electrolyte disturbances, ischemia, or toxic drug levels, particularly digitalis (see Chapter 21).

ATRIAL CONDUCTION PATHWAY

JUNCTION

VENTRICULAR CONDUCTION PATHWAY

177

One of the primary effects of junctional rhythms is a decreased cardiac output resulting from ineffective depolarization of the atria and loss of atrial contraction **(atrial kick)**.

What IS AV Junctional (Nodal) Rhythm? 40 – 60 Bpm

Because the junctional tissue is anatomically located between the atrial and ventricular conduction pathways, impulses that originate in this area may conduct several ways.

Redrawn from Paul, Hebra: *The nurse's guide to cardiac rhythm interpretation,* Philadelphia, 1998, Saunders, p. 111.

Impulses may originate in the AV tissue and conduct down the bundle of His, right and left bundle branches, Purkinje fibers, and ventricular cells, resulting in no P wave and a normal width QRS complex (i.e., less than ~~0.12~~ seconds). 0.10 Sec

Impulses may originate in the AV tissue and conduct in a backward **(retrograde)** fashion through the atria, resulting in an inverted P wave in lead II, which normally has positive P waves. The inverted P wave may occur before the QRS, indicating retrograde atrial depolarization occurred before ventricular depolarization, or the inverted P wave may occur after the QRS, indicating the retrograde atrial depolarization occurred after the ventricular depolarization.

Impulses may originate in AV tissue, which results in an upright P wave occurring before the QRS; however, the PR interval is shorter than normal (less than 0.20 seconds).

The intrinsic rate for the AV node is between 40 and 60 bpm. If the SA node is damaged or diseased to the point at which it will not fire or initiate conduction at a rate greater than the inherent rate of the AV node, the AV node simply takes over the conduction system at that point. If the SA node recovers, the AV node will relinquish its pace-making activities.

What You NEED TO KNOW

Generally, there is no treatment for a junctional rhythm if the rate is sufficient for cardiac output. Transvenous pacing may be necessary for this purpose if it is anticipated that the SA node will not recover and perform its duties.

The patient may be given an antidysrhythmic drug (e.g., atropine) if the slower rate (**bradycardia**) results in symptoms such as chest pain, shortness of breath (**dyspnea**), or decreased level of consciousness.

Patients with AV junctional tissue disturbances should be observed closely for degeneration to more serious rhythms, such as heart blocks or ventricular escape rhythms. If the AV node fails as a pacemaker, the inherent rate of the ventricular pacemaker is fewer than 40 bpm.

If treatment is effective, the patient will sustain sufficient cardiac output and, if possible, experience restoration of the SA node as the primary pacemaker.

What You DO

When working with a patient with a junctional rhythm, you should do the following:
- Identify the dysrhythmia as junctional (i.e., nodal) in origin as distinguished from sinus bradycardia or advanced heart block. Document it and notify the health care provider if onset is sudden.
- Observe the monitor carefully for any new ectopic activity, such as premature ventricular contractions (PVCs).

TAKE HOME POINTS

If a rhythm meets the criteria for being defined as junctional (i.e., no P wave, inverted P wave before or after the QRS, or a short PR interval with a normal QRS complex and a rate between 40 and 60 bpm), it is referred to as a junctional rhythm or a junctional escape rhythm.

- Offending drugs, such as a digitalis glycoside (e.g., digoxin) or a group IA antidysrhythmic (e.g., quinidine), should be withdrawn promptly. The slower heart rate makes the conduction system more vulnerable to other pacemakers in the cardiac muscle, such as irritable foci in the ventricles that can result in ventricular tachycardias.
- The sudden occurrence of a nodal rhythm when the SA node has previously initiated the cardiac cycle is generally a sign of downward deterioration or displacement of the conduction system. Heart blocks or ventricular dysrhythmias may quickly follow.

TAKE HOME POINTS

Particular attention must be paid to the ECG tracings when the patient has had a heart attack. Inflammation or swelling of heart tissue encasing the conduction system can cause temporary dysfunction, although permanent damage may be evident if oxygen is not restored in time.

To determine whether a rhythm is junctional (nodal), you should observe for the following:

- **Rate:** Between 40 and 60 bpm.
- **Rhythm:** Regular
- **PR interval:** Abnormal P waves may be inverted or absent (Intervals may occur before, after, or within the QRS complex. PR interval < 0.12 seconds if P wave is in the QRS; if not, it is not measurable.)
- **QRS:** Normal
- **QT:** Measurable, within normal limits

If the rate is less than 50 per minute, be alert for changes that signal cardiovascular insufficiency (e.g., chest pain, shortness of breath, change in level of consciousness, dizziness).

- If the patient is taking a drug that is intended to lower heart rate, such as digitalis glycosides (digoxin), consult with the prescribing health care provider before continued drug administration.

Do You UNDERSTAND?

DIRECTIONS: Fill in the blanks.

1. A rhythm is considered junctional when _____ _____ _____.

2. When the AV node works as a _____ to generate an impulse, it has the ability to generate impulses at a rate of _____ bpm.

3. In the following strips, locate the P waves.

a.

b.

Inverted P waves

b.

Upright P   Upright P   Inverted P   Upright P   Inverted P   Upright P   Upright P

a.

Answers:

c.

What IS a Premature Junctional Contraction?

A *premature junctional contraction* (PJC) occurs when an irritable area in the junctional tissue generates an impulse before the next SA node–initiated beat, resulting in an early beat. This beat has the features of a junctional beat and occurs sooner than the next normal beat would have occurred.

If the PJCs are infrequent, no treatment is necessary. Frequently occurring PJCs may mean increasing ischemia or irritability. Frequent PJCs may result in the sudden onset of a junctional tachycardia. Junctional tachycardias begin within or near the AV node and are considered to be an automatic focus tachycardia, meaning an irritable cell within the AV junctional tissue fires repetitively to generate the tachycardia. Automatic focus tachycardias do not respond to electrical car-

No P waves

c.

Answer:

dioversion. The treatment of automatic focus tachycardias, including junctional tachycardias, is medication such as β-blockers, calcium channel blockers, or amiodarone to suppress the irritable focus. If treatment is effective, it is expected that the patient's rhythm will be restored to normal sinus rhythm (NSR) or the rate will be controlled. Often, the patient is not aware of PJCs unless they occur frequently or cause palpitations.

Redrawn from Paul, Hebra: *The nurse's guide to cardiac rhythm interpretation,* Philadelphia, 1998, Saunders, p. 108.

What You NEED TO KNOW

If the PJCs occur infrequently, no treatment is necessary. Frequently occurring PJCs may indicate increasing ischemia or irritability. If frequent PJCs result in runs of tachycardias, intravenous antidysrhythmic medications may be necessary. If treatment is effective, it is expected that the patient's rhythm will be restored to normal sinus rhythm (NSR) without premature beats or more serious dysrhythmias. Often the patient is not aware of a PJC unless they occur frequently or cause palpitations.

When working with a patient with PJC, you should do the following:

- Identify the premature contraction as junctional in nature as distinguished from the more serious PVC. (Remember that PVCs have QRS complexes that are wider than normal [greater than 0.11 seconds].)
- Notify the health care provider if frequency increases or patient becomes symptomatic.
- Give drugs as prescribed and monitor effectiveness.

 TAKE HOME POINTS

To determine whether a beat is a PJC, you should observe for the following:
- **Rate:** Underlying rhythm
- **Rhythm:** Irregular because of the early beat (PJC)
- **P wave (associated with PJC):** May be absent, inverted before or after the QRS complex; PR interval may be short (< 0.11 seconds)
- **QRS complex:** Within normal limits (< 0.11 seconds)

Do You UNDERSTAND?

DIRECTIONS: Cite the characteristics of a PJC.
1. Rate: _____
2. P wave: _____
3. QRS: _____
4. Rhythm: _____

DIRECTIONS: Unscramble the letters in the word jumble to fill in the blanks.
5. If PJCs increase in frequency, there is a possibility that _____ dysrhythmias may arise. *(cetrvniluar)*
6. A PJC causes the rhythm to be _____ because the beat occurs earlier than the next normal beat. *(guirrlear)*

What IS a Junctional Tachycardia?

By definition, a tachycardia is a rhythm with a rate greater than 100 bpm. A *junctional tachycardia* is a rhythm that fits the criteria for being junctional (i.e., no P waves with a normal QRS complex, inverted P waves before or after the QRS complex in a lead where Ps are normally upright, or short PR intervals with a normal QRS complex) and has a rate greater than 100 bpm.

Redrawn from Paul, Hebra: *The nurse's guide to cardiac rhythm interpretation,* Philadelphia, 1998, Saunders, p. 83.

Answers: 1. that of the underlying rhythm; 2. not identified or occurs after or within QRS complexes; 3. should be within normal limits (but may be widened if there is an intraventricular conduction delay); 4. irregular, because of early beat PJC; 5. ventricular; 6. irregular.

SVT/PSVT

Often in tachycardias, rates get so fast that it becomes difficult to identify P waves and analyze the rhythm strip. Because the QRS is usually the most easily identified waveform in the patient with a cardiac history, the QRS complex width can be measured and determined to be normal or abnormal. If the QRS complex is within normal limits (i.e., less than 0.12 seconds), conduction through the ventricles has occurred normally, and the rhythm originated *above* the ventricles.

A rhythm can be classified as supraventricular when the exact origin of the rhythm is uncertain, when it is difficult to identify P waves, and when the QRS complex is of normal width. A supraventricular tachycardia (SVT) originates above the ventricles and has a rate greater than 100 bpm. These rhythms often start suddenly and end abruptly; thus, the term *paroxysmal.* Paroxysmal supraventricular tachycardia (PSVT) includes atrial tachycardias and junctional tachycardias; however, the term is used when the origin of the tachycardia cannot be specifically identified.

What You NEED TO KNOW

It is important to understand that although junctional tachycardias originate above the ventricles and are classified as a type of SVT, the mechanism for causing the junctional tachycardia is an irritable (automatic) focus. As discussed in the section earlier on premature junctional contractions, automatic focus tachycardias do not respond to cardioversion. They should be treated with medications that suppress the irritable cell.

A reentry of the conduction stimulus through the AV node or through a concealed bypass tract is responsible for more than 90% of all PSVTs. Others may be caused by any catecholamine, neurotransmitter release (e.g., epinephrine), or sympathetic response provoked by such events as anxiety, caffeine intake, hypoglycemia, fear, stress, or digitalis toxicity.

If the cause of the catecholamine release can be determined and controlled, the PSVT may end as abruptly as it began without treatment. However, if PSVT is sustained, the health care provider should intervene based on institutional protocols. Advanced Cardiac Life Support (ACLS) guidelines suggest attempting to establish a specific diagnosis based on a 12-lead ECG and clinical information. Vagal maneuvers such as carotid sinus massage, forceful coughing, diving reflex, or Valsalva maneuver may induce reflex vagal (10th cranial nerve) stimulation and either slow the heart rate or interrupt the rhythm. Note: In many institutions, carotid sinus massage is only performed by physicians. It is essential to follow institutional protocols for interventions. If there is no response to these attempts to include reflex vagal stimulation, cardioversion may be used to restore normal sinus rhythm and rate in tachycardias that have a reentry mechanism. The antidysrhythmic adenosine may also be given by IV if carotid massage is unsuccessful.

If PSVT occurs repeatedly, drug intervention with digitalis glycosides (e.g., digoxin), class IA antidysrhythmics (e.g., quinidine), or Group II antidysrhythmic (e.g., propranolol) may be required.

If the PSVT is caused by atrial fibrillation or atrial flutter, the patient should be evaluated for clinical stability, and the duration of the PSVT (either longer or shorter than 48 hours) should be determined. Unstable patients should be treated immediately with cardioversion. Antidysrhythmic agents are used to control the rate and convert the rhythm in stable patients. The American Heart Association's ACLS guidelines promote anticoagulation for these patients.

Most patients are immediately aware of PSVT because of the rapid heart action, a fluttering sensation in the chest, and light-headedness. The dizziness occurs because of the reduced stroke volume (the result of shortened ventricular filling time) with the rapid rate and the small subsequent quantities of blood perfusing the cerebral tissue. Patients are very uncomfortable and will seek immediate relief.

If the tachycardia is sustained, cardiac output may drop. With a decrease in cardiac output and an increase in myocardial oxygen consumption, the patient may experience angina or myocardial ischemia.

PSVT has an abrupt onset and may also subside abruptly without treatment. The expected outcome is that the heart rate will return to NSR without complications.

> ⚠ If the duration of the atrial fibrillation is longer than 48 hours, caution should be used when using agents that convert the rhythm in patients not adequately anticoagulated because of the possibility of embolic problems.

What You DO

When working with a patient with junctional tachycardia, you should do the following:

- Remember that the onset of PSVT will trigger the high-rate alarm, at which time you should assess the patient, verify the rapid pulse rate, and document it.

- Notify the health care provider immediately, and observe the patient for signs of chest pain or heart failure.
- Obtain the vital signs.
- If the patient remains stable, keep in mind that vagal maneuvers or intravenous drugs (e.g., adenosine) may be used to interrupt the rapid rhythm.
- If the patient becomes unstable (e.g., hypotensive) or displays symptoms, such as shortness of breath, chest pain, or changes in level of consciousness, immediate cardioversion is indicated.
- A brief trial of medications may be considered before cardioversion, and sedation should be considered for patients needing cardioversion.

LIFE SPAN

SVT can occur in neonates and children because of immature sympathetic nervous system (SNS) development. Although most SVTs in young patients will resolve without medical intervention, their overall physiologic status should be closely monitored. Certain drugs that are used to treat adult SVTs may be lethal in neonates and very young children.

Do You UNDERSTAND?

DIRECTIONS: **Check which of the following descriptions pertains to PSVT.**

1. _____ a. Normal cardiac rate with early contractions, abnormal P-waves, and regular rhythm.

_____ b. Cardiac rate of 100 to 140 bpm, regular P waves, compensatory pauses, and regular QRS complexes.

_____ c. Rates greater than 150 bpm, abnormally shaped and sometimes buried P waves, narrow QRS complexes, and regular rhythm.

_____ d. Rate greater than 250 bpm, irregular P waves, widened QRS complexes, irregular rhythm.

Redrawn from Paul, Hebra: *The nurse's guide to cardiac rhythm interpretation*, Philadelphia, 1998, Saunders, p. 61.

TAKE HOME POINTS

The term PSVT is used when medical personnel are unable to specifically identify the origin of the tachycardia because of lack of clearly identifiable P waves.

PSVT can be distinguished from ventricular tachycardia because the QRS complex is not wider than normal. (A normal QRS complex indicates the rhythm originated above the ventricles because ventricular conduction was normal.)

To determine whether a rhythm is PSVT, you should observe for the following:

- **Rate:** Usually greater than 150 bpm
- **P waves:** Difficult to identify; rates are fast and P waves may be hidden or buried in T waves (If the tachycardia is sudden in onset [i.e., paroxysmal], you can find P waves by looking at the very first beat in the run. There may be a visible P wave with the first beat.)
- **Rhythm:** Regular
- **PR interval:** P wave may be hidden in the QRS or sitting on top of T waves
- **QRS:** Usually normal width
- **QT:** Measurable, within normal limits

Answer: 1. c.

Redrawn from Paul, Hebra: *The nurse's guide to cardiac rhythm interpretation,* Philadelphia, 1998, Saunders, p. 102.

DIRECTIONS: **Provide the answers to the following questions.**

2. When taking vital signs, the nurse notes that Mr. Jones has an apical rate of 120 bpm and Mr. Smith has an apical rate of 200 bpm. Both men are experiencing some type of what?

   _____

3. The nurse then observes the telemetry monitors to view their cardiac rhythms. To determine the probable origin of their rhythms, what observation should the nurse make first?

   _____

   _____

4. Based on these observations, what are the two rhythms?
   Mr. Jones has _____.
   Mr. Smith has _____.

DIRECTIONS: **Complete the crossword puzzle.**

Across

1. In atrial dysrhythmias, stimulus is not from this node.
3. Increased heart rates require greater _____ consumption by the heart muscle.
4. Pressure may be applied to the globe of this organ by a physician to slow the heart rate.
7. 170 to 250 times per minute.
8. Any type can provoke general catecholamine release.

Down

1. Paroxysmal.
2. PSVT rhythm is _____.
5. Can refer to both onset and termination.
6. PSVT may be caused by this.

What IS an Accelerated Junctional Rhythm?

An accelerated rhythm is one that is faster than the inherent rate for the pacemaker of origin but not fast enough to be a tachycardia. An *accelerated junctional rhythm* is a junctional rhythm with a rate between 60 and 100 bpm. (Remember, the normal rate for a junctional rhythm is 40 to 60 bpm.)

What You NEED TO KNOW

- If the SA node is suppressed and the AV junctional tissues act as the compensatory pacemaker, the inherent rate is 40 to 60 bpm.
- Junctional rhythms with rates in excess of 60 bpm are accelerated junctional rhythms and are commonly caused by digitalis toxicity.
- Treatment of accelerated junctional rhythms is aimed at identifying the cause. If the rate is fast enough to be considered an accelerated junctional rhythm, the rhythm may support cardiac output and would not be suppressed unless there is evidence that the SA node will assume the responsibility as primary pacemaker.

 Be prepared to assist with emergency interventions if patient becomes unstable.

TAKE HOME POINTS

- **Rate:** Greater than 60 bpm but less than 100 bpm
- **Rhythm:** Regular
- **P waves:** Absent with a normal-width QRS complex, inverted in lead II before or after a normal width QRS complex; PR interval may be shorter than normal (< 0.12 seconds)
- **QRS complex:** Should be normal (< 0.12 seconds); may be wider with an intraventricular-conduction delay

What You DO

When working with a patient with an accelerated junctional rhythm, you should do the following:
- Monitor the heart rate.
- Assess the patient for adequacy of perfusion.
- Assess for the absence of chest pain and an adequate level of consciousness.
- Check the patient for shortness of breath.
- Determine that there is no hypotension.
- Monitor serum digoxin levels and levels of other antidysrhythmic drugs.

Do You UNDERSTAND?

DIRECTIONS: **Examine the sample ECG strip, and answer the following questions.**

Redrawn from Paul, Hebra: *The nurse's guide to cardiac rhythm interpretation,* Philadelphia, 1998, Saunders, p. 113.

1. Why would this strip be recognized as a junctional rhythm?

_____

_____

2. Why would it be called an accelerated junctional rhythm?

_____

3. Where are the P waves?

_____

_____

References

Aehlert B: *ECGs made easy,* ed 2, St Louis, 2002, Mosby.

American Heart Association: *Advanced cardiac life support provider manual,* Dallas, 1997, American Heart Association.

Conover M: *Understanding electrocardiography,* ed 7, St Louis, 1996, Mosby.

Cummins RO, editor: *Textbook of advanced cardiac life support,* Dallas, 1997, American Heart Association.

Ehrat K: *The art of EKG interpretation: a self-instruction text,* Dubuque, 1997, Kendall/Hunt.

Hartshorn JC, Sole ML, Lamborn ML: *Introduction to critical care nursing,* ed 3, Philadelphia, 2001, Saunders.

Hellstedt LF: *Sorting out supraventricular tachycardias: critical care choices 98,* Springhouse, Penn, 1998, Springhouse.

Paul S, Hebra J: *The nurse's guide to cardiac rhythm interpretation: implications for patient care,* Philadelphia, 1998, Saunders.

Singh BN: Antiarrhythmic actions or amiodarone: a profile of a paradoxical agent, *Am J Cardiol* 78(4A):41, 1996.

NCLEX® Review

1. Mrs. Anthony was admitted with an accelerated junctional tachycardia. In obtaining Mrs. Anthony's drug history, which medication should alert the health care provider as to a possible cause for this dysrhythmia?
   1 Stool softener
   2 Sedative
   3 Antihypertensive
   4 Digitalis glycoside

2. The conduction system of the heart includes inherent pacemakers at varying locations. Which of the following ECG tracing descriptions might the health care practitioner observe if the atrioventricular node is the primary pacemaker?
   1 Absence of P waves and a ventricular rate less than 40 bpm
   2 Abnormally shaped QRS complexes
   3 Abnormal or inverted P waves and a ventricular rate between 40 and 60 bpm
   4 Depressed ST segments

3. Mr. Collins develops paroxysmal supraventricular tachycardia. What initial therapy might be attempted?
   1 Cardioversion
   2 Intravenous atropine
   3 Intravenous epinephrine
   4 Vagal stimulation

4. All the following are indicators of junctional beats *except:*
   1 PR interval less than 0.12 seconds
   2 No P wave
   3 PR interval greater than 0.20 seconds
   4 Retrograde or inverted P wave in lead II

5. In paroxysmal supraventricular tachycardia, cardiac output is reduced because of:
   1 Wide QRS complexes
   2 Shortened diastolic filling time
   3 Increased stroke volume
   4 Slowed heart rate

6. A junctional rhythm with a ventricular rate exceeding 60 bpm but less than 100 bpm is referred to as:
   1 Ventricular escape rhythm
   2 Junctional tachycardia
   3 Bradycardia
   4 Accelerated junctional rhythm

7. Supraventricular tachycardias may occur in what group(s) of people because of immature sympathetic nervous system development?
   1 Teenagers and young adults
   2 Neonates and children
   3 Mature adults
   4 Infants and teenagers

8. The health care provider is assessing a rhythm strip and having difficulty identifying P waves. The QRS complexes are less than 0.12 seconds wide. The ventricular rate is 122. The rhythm strip most probably should be identified as:
   1 Ventricular tachycardia
   2 A junctional rhythm
   3 Sinus tachycardia
   4 Supraventricular tachycardia

9. A junctional rhythm with retrograde atrial conduction would be indicated by which of the following?
   1 PR interval greater than 0.28 seconds
   2 PR interval less than 0.12 seconds
   3 P waves upright in lead II
   4 P waves negative in lead II

10. Which of the following therapies might be used to treat supraventricular tachycardia?
    1 Atropine
    2 Adenosine
    3 Cardioversion
    4 Vagal maneuvers

NCLEX® Review Answers

1. 4 Digoxin, a digitalis glycoside, is often the culprit in initiating junctional tachycardia. Additional doses of digoxin could be lethal in this situation. A stool softener is given to decrease a vagal response that could cause sinus bradycardia or heart block. A sedative usually slows the heart rate rather than increases it. An antihypertensive drug, which is a centrally acting sympatholytically, reduces cerebral sympatholytic outflow, thereby decreasing sympathetic responses (decreasing heart rate) and peripheral resistance.

2. 3 A junctional rhythm may have abnormal or inverted P waves. The inherent rate for the atrioventricular node is 40 to 60 bpm. Absence of P waves with a ventricular rate of less than 40 is slower than a typical junctional rhythm. In a junctional rhythm, the QRS complexes should be less than 0.12 seconds wide and shaped normally. In a junctional rhythm, the ST segments are normally isoelectric, unless there is some ischemia.

3. 4 Vagal maneuvers are used initially to slow the heart rate and allow the sinus node to resume pacemaker activities; however, if this is not successful, cardioversion is used. Cardioversion may be used if the patient is unstable or the rate is greater than 150 bpm. Intravenous atropine is administered to increase heart rate. Intravenous epinephrine is a sympathomimetic medication and will increase heart rate.

4. 3 A PR interval greater than 0.2 seconds indicates a first-degree atrioventricular block. Junctional beats may have P waves and short PR intervals (less than 0.12 seconds). Junctional beats may have no P waves. A junctional rhythm may have inverted P waves in lead II.

5. 2 Cardiac output is a result of stroke volume times heart rate. In tachycardias, the increased heart rate shortens diastolic filling time, thus decreasing stroke volume and cardiac output. Wide QRS complexes indicate slowed conduction through the ventricles. Increased stroke volume would occur when there is adequate diastolic filling time, normal afterload, and appropriate contractility. Heart rate is one of the components in the cardiac output formula. Slowed rates decrease cardiac output if the stroke volume does not increase.

6. 4 The definition of an accelerated rhythm is a rhythm that is faster than the inherent rate but not fast enough to be a tachycardia. An accelerated junctional rhythm has a rate between 60 and 100 bpm. A ventricular escape rhythm has a rate between 20 and 40 bpm. A junctional tachycardia has a rate greater than 100 bpm. A bradycardia has a rate less than 60 bpm.

7. 2 Neonates and children have not developed a mature sympathetic nervous system and therefore may experience supraventricular tachycardias. Teenagers, young adults, and mature adults should have a mature sympathetic nervous system.

8. 4 A supraventricular tachycardia has a rate greater than 100 with difficulty identifying P waves and the QRS complexes are normal (< 0.12 seconds wide). A ventricular tachycardia will have a rate greater than 100 with no apparent P waves; however, the QRS complexes will be wide (> 0.12 seconds). A junctional rhythm will have a rate between 40 and 60 bpm. A sinus tachycardia will have a rate greater than 100 with a normal-width QRS; however, in a sinus tachycardia, P waves should be identifiable.

9. **4** Negative P waves in lead II indicate retrograde conduction and are indicative of a junctional rhythm. A PR interval greater than 0.28 seconds would be indicative of a first-degree atrioventricular block. A junctional rhythm may have a PR interval less than 0.12 seconds; however, if retrograde conduction occurs, the P wave will be inverted in lead II. In a junctional rhythm with retrograde conduction, the P wave is inverted, not upright, in lead II.

10. **1** Atropine is used to treat symptomatic bradycardias. Adenosine may be used to treat narrow complex tachycardias. Cardioversion is used in supraventricular tachycardias when the patient is symptomatic or rates exceed 150 bpm, usually after vagal maneuvers are used. Vagal maneuvers are initially used to slow a supraventricular tachycardia in an attempt to allow the sinus node to regain control.

Notes

Chapter 11
Practice Strips

Please analyze and identify information for each of the following ECG strips.

Strip 1   Rate:_____ Rhythm: _____ P wave: _____

PR interval:_____ QRS:_____

Rhythm interpretation:_____

Strip 2   Rate:_____ Rhythm:_____ P wave: _____

PR interval:_____ QRS:_____

Rhythm interpretation:_____

Strip 3   Rate:_____ Rhythm:_____P wave:_____

PR interval:_____ QRS: _____

Rhythm interpretation:_____

Premature Ventricular Contractions

What You WILL LEARN

After reading this chapter, you will know how to do the following:

✔ Describe the characteristics of a premature ventricular contraction (PVC).

✔ Name two causes of PVCs.

✔ Describe what you assess when determining PVCs on an ECG.

What IS a Premature Ventricular Contraction?

A *premature ventricular contraction* (PVC) is an ectopic beat originating in either the left or the right ventricle. It comes early in the cardiac cycle, before the next expected beat (prematurely), and it occurs in the presence of an underlying rhythm, usually a sinus rhythm.

What You NEED TO KNOW

The PVC appears as a premature beat with a wide QRS, no P wave, and a long pause after it. There is no P wave because the SA node does not initiate the beat. The pause is called a compensatory pause; it occurs because the ventricle is in a refractory phase after the PVC, and it is unable to respond to any stimulus until the next beat.

The QRS is wide because conduction does not travel down the normal pathway. The PVC takes longer to get through the ventricular myocardium when it has to go from one cell to another, instead of staying "on track" in the cells of the conduction system.

PVCs hit prematurely—before the ventricle has had a chance to completely fill with blood. As a result, the ventricle must pump less than the normal amount of blood (**stroke volume**) with that beat. The PVC may not be felt by the patient or it may be perceived as a *skipped beat*. It may be described as a little thump in the chest and may be accompanied by a perceived need to take a deep breath. However, it is really an *extra beat* that is weakly perfused, and an apical and radial pulse deficit may be noted. The beat after a PVC is often stronger because the ventricle has a chance to *overfill* after the compensatory pause.

PVCs are caused by ventricular irritability which may be due to sympathetic nervous system (SNS) stimulation by caffeine, drugs, or emotional stress. Also, changes in the excitability threshold of the ventricular tissue can be caused by digitalis toxicity, hypoxia, hypokalemia, or myocardial ischemia. Treating the underlying cause is the most important nursing intervention in breaking the rhythm.

Some PVCs are benign, and others are more dangerous. PVCs occur in many healthy persons for no apparent reason. In general, PVCs are only dangerous if they decrease the cardiac output or if they lead to more lethal dysrhythmias.

 In a patient with acute heart disease or lung disease, PVCs can be a warning of increased ventricular irritability that could lead to ventricular tachycardia or ventricular fibrillation.

What You DO

Recognizing a PVC

The most distinguishing characteristic of the PVC is the wide and bizarre QRS that stands out in the midst of an otherwise mundane rhythm.

Characteristics

Rate: The underlying rate is normal, fast, or slow.

Rhythm: The underlying rhythm can be regular, but the PVC disrupts the regularity by firing prematurely.

P wave: None. May appear as a small wave very close to or after the PVC, yet unrelated to it.

QRS: Complex is wide (greater than 0.12 seconds), premature, bizarrely shaped.

TAKE HOME POINTS

PVC may be a warning sign of a more serious ventricular dysrhythmia.

LIFE SPAN

In the middle-aged adult, PVCs may need further follow-up for possible coronary artery disease. PVCs are more frequent in the older patient, especially those with long-standing pulmonary disease, cardiac disease, or both.

ST segments and T waves: Both may be elevated or sloped in opposite directions of the QRS.

Compensatory pause: Interval between the R waves of the normal beats surrounding the PVC (the one immediately before and after the PVC) should be equal to the intervals between three normal beats without a PVC.

The QRS in the following rhythm strip is 0.16 second in width. (Remember, the PVC ends at the J point.) In the PVC in this strip, the ST segment is elevated, and the T wave is tall. The direction of the QRS is negative, which is the opposite direction of the underlying rhythm.

A PVC sticks out like a sore thumb and is usually the easiest ectopic beat to recognize. If there is any doubt whether a beat is a PVC, it is sometimes helpful to look at it in a second lead.

Compensatory
pause

CULTURE

Blacks have a higher incidence of coronary artery disease, hypertension, and sudden death; therefore they are more prone to PVCs.

Do You UNDERSTAND?

DIRECTIONS: Circle all the possible characteristics of the PVC.

No P wave	Compensatory pause
P wave premature	Flat ST segments
PR greater than 0.20	ST opposite of normal beats
No QRS	T wave opposite of normal beats
QRS wide	QRS premature

Answers: **No P wave, QRS wide, Compensatory pause, QRS premature, ST opposite of normal beats, T wave opposite of normal beats.**

What ARE the Patterns of PVCs?

PVCs come in various forms depending on where they originate in the ventricle and the pattern in which they fire. Patterns of PVCs include unifocal, multifocal, couplet, bigeminy and trigeminy, and R-on-T phenomenon.

TAKE HOME POINTS

- PVCs may also be found in normal, healthy individuals. The cause should be investigated to rule out heart disease.
- Quick fixes for PVCs. 1) Check pulse oximetry—administer oxygen if Spo$_2$ < 92%. 2) Check serum potassium. Administer supplemental potassium (with physician order) if K < 3.5.

What You NEED TO KNOW

How do you know which PVCs are dangerous and need to be treated? Generally, occasional, unifocal, isolated PVCs are fairly common and harmless. All others should be closely evaluated because they may lead to more lethal dysrhythmias.

Unifocal PVCs

Unifocal or uniform PVCs are premature ventricular beats that look the same (see above strip). They are caused by a single, irritable focus in the ventricles. The PVC in the above strip is a simple, isolated, unifocal PVC.

TAKE HOME POINTS

Uniform, isolated, infrequent PVCs are common and do not usually need to be treated. An increasing number of PVCs suggests increasing ventricular irritability and a need for closer attention.

Multifocal PVCs

Redrawn from Phipps, Sands, Marek: *Medical-surgical nursing: concepts and clinical practice,* ed 6, St Louis, 1999, Mosby, p. 673.

• Multifocal PVCs indicate a more serious level of ventricular irritability than unifocal PVCs, and they are more likely to lead to more serious dysrhythmias.
• Always check potassium and magnesium levels.

Multifocal or multiform PVCs are those with different shapes—they do not all look alike because they are coming from different locations in the ventricles (see above strip). As you can imagine, multifocal PVCs indicate a more serious level of ventricular irritability than unifocal PVCs, and they are more likely to lead to more serious dysrhythmias (e.g., ventricular fibrillation).

Couplets

Redrawn from Paul, Hebra: *The nurse's guide to cardiac rhythm interpretation,* Philadelphia, 1998, Saunders, p. 131.

Although couplets are not usually dangerous, they can suggest ventricular irritability and may eventually lead to ventricular tachycardia.

Couplets are paired PVCs or two PVCs in a row; they could be called "kissing cousins" (see above strip). They may be unifocal (as in the top rhythm strip); they may also be multifocal (as in the bottom rhythm strip). Like multifocal PVCs, couplets are an indicator of advanced ventricular irritability. When PVCs occur three or more in a row, it is called ventricular tachycardia (see Chapter 13).

Ventricular Bigeminy and Trigeminy

Bigeminy
PVC every other beat

Trigeminy
PVC every third beat

There are times when PVCs fall in a very regular and predictable pattern. (They have a "regular irregularity" about them.) Perhaps in palpating a patient's heartbeat, you have felt the pattern skip every other beat or skip a beat after two normal heartbeats. This pattern may be *ventricular bigeminy or ventricular trigeminy.*

Bigeminy occurs when every other beat is a PVC; in other words, there will be one normal beat and one PVC. Ventricular trigeminy is two normal beats and a PVC. Ventricular quadrigeminy is indicated by a PVC every fourth beat. These rhythms are not usually treated, but they are monitored closely.

R-on-T Phenomenon

Redrawn from Ignatavicius, Workman, Mishler: *Medical-surgical nursing across the health care continuum,* ed 2, Philadelphia, 1995, Saunders, p. 852.

TAKE HOME POINTS

When PVCs become increasingly more frequent, multifocal, or coupled, or when they fall close to the T wave, they should be taken more seriously as a sign that DANGEROUS, LIFE-THREATENING RHYTHMS, such as ventricular tachycardia and ventricular fibrillation, are possible. Therefore emergency drugs and a defibrillator should be immediately accessible.

The R-on-T phenomenon type of PVC can be potentially dangerous to the patient. This danger does not have to do with the size or shape of the PVC; rather with its location in the cardiac cycle. The QRS of the PVC is very close to or on the T wave (repolarization) of the previous beat. The last section of the T wave is considered the vulnerable (refractory) period of the heart's cycle. Any stimulus during this stage, when the electrolytes are trying to reorganize themselves, can set the heart into a run of life-threatening ventricular tachycardia.

Causes of PVCs (Acute)

Acute, treatable causes of PVCs include hypokalemia, hypoxemia, hypomagnesemia, hypocalcemia, acidemia, hypoxemia, stress, fever, and drugs. They may be remembered by the following mnemonic device:

HANK	= Hypoxemia
AND	= Acidemia
HARRY	= Hypokalemia
HAVE	= Hypocalcemia
DEPRESSED	= Drugs (digoxin)
ENLARGED	= Epinephrine (stress, emotions, fever, heart failure)
HEARTS	= Hypomagnesemia

Chronic Causes of PVCs

There are certain chronic diseases of the heart in which PVCs are common and expected. Patients with these diseases may already be on oral antidysrhythmic drugs and are therefore not treated unless symptomatic. If treatment is indicated, lidocaine or amiodarone may be used.

Condition	Cause
Heart failure	Fluid build up in lungs; heart has to pump a heavier load and push against increased resistance
Myocarditis	Inflammation of the heart causes swelling and compression of chambers, thus decreasing filling
Arteriosclerotic heart disease	Hardening of cardiac arteries decreases blood supply to the heart
Ventricular aneurysm	Weakening of ventricular wall leads to weakening of the heart pump
Cardiomegaly	Enlarged heart will not contract as easily

TAKE HOME POINTS

Some patients have chronic ventricular ectopy with which the health care provider may be perfectly comfortable and elect not to treat. Be sure to consult with the health care provider to determine whether the patient has preexisting ectopy, which does not need to be treated.

What You DO

When working with a patient with PVCs, you should do the following:

- Assess the patient for signs and symptoms of decreased cardiac output (e.g., hypotension, light-headedness).
- Assess the patient's pulse to see whether PVCs are perfusing. The apical pulse may be greater than the radial pulse because the PVCs may not perfuse as strongly. The PVCs may not be felt at all or may be described as "skipped beats."
- Most PVCs do not require treatment unless they lead to ventricular tachycardia. They should however be considered "warning signs" to look for, and their causes should be treated. Monitor the patient's oxygen level with pulse oximetry. Place patient on oxygen if necessary.
- Monitor serum electrolyte levels (potassium, magnesium, calcium), and supplement if necessary. Be especially astute in patients with vomiting and/or diarrhea who have been NPO (nothing by mouth).
- Monitor digoxin level for toxicity and acid base level for acidosis.
- Assess sympathetic nervous system (SNS) causes (e.g., stress, pain, anger, fear, fever), and remove the cause if possible.
- Consider whether the patient could be in heart failure. The heart will become irritable when overstretched.
- Evaluate possibility of side effects from drugs such as caffeine, nicotine, aminophylline, dopamine, epinephrine.
- Assess chest pain to rule out acute coronary syndrome. (If indicated, obtain 12-lead ECG.)
- Document the presence and type of PVCs on the rhythm strip. Include the name of the underlying rhythm. For example, "sinus rhythm at 70 beats/min with occasional, isolated, unifocal PVCs."
- Become familiar with your patient's history to know whether PVCs are commonly seen in the patient.
- Notify the health care provider if PVCs are a new finding.
- Prophylactic treatment is no longer recommended in the setting of acute coronary syndrome. Treatment is instead directed at oxygenation, relief of pain, and coronary reperfusion. Drugs such as nitrates, thrombolytic agents, platelet inhibitors, β-blockers, and narcotics are used, along with invasive coronary reperfusion intervention.

TAKE HOME POINTS

Advanced Cardiac Life Support (ACLS) protocols do not recommend that PVCs be routinely treated. The cause of the ventricular irritability should be investigated and treated instead.

Do You UNDERSTAND?

DIRECTIONS: **Match the key words in column A with the types of PVCs in column B.**

Coluwmn A	Column B
1. _____ All look the same	a. Trigeminy
2. _____ One beat, one PVC	b. Multifocal
3. _____ All look different	c. Bigeminy
4. _____ Four PVCs in a row	d. Unifocal
5. _____ Too close to the T wave	e. Ventricular tachycardia
6. _____ Two beats, one PVC	f. R on T
7. _____ Low oxygen level	g. Anger
8. _____ Bronchodilating drug	h. Hypokalemia
9. _____ Rage	i. Stress
10. _____ pH of blood goes down	j. Digoxin
11. _____ Low potassium	k. Hypoxemia
12. _____ May cause toxicity	l. Acidemia
13. _____ Elevated temperature	m. MI
14. _____ Myocardial infarction	n. Fever
15. _____ Sympathetic stimulation	o. Epinephrine

DIRECTIONS: **Indicate which answers are correct and which are incorrect.**

16. Which actions should be taken upon noticing an increase in the frequency of PVCs?

_____ Assess the patient

_____ Check potassium and magnesium levels

_____ Check digitalis level

_____ Assess oxygenation status

_____ Review medication record

www.cpr-ecc.american
heart.org
www.usfca.edu/fac-staff/
ritter/public_html/
fourekg.htm
www.wices.com/
icescardiac4.htm
www.ace.cr/newaclsguide
lines.htm

References

Aehlert B: *ECGs made easy,* ed 2, St Louis, 2002, Mosby.

American Heart Association: *Advanced cardiac life support provider manual,* Dallas, 2001, American Heart Association.

Bloomquist J, Love M: Cardiovascular assessment and diagnostic procedures. In Urden L, Stacy K, editors: *Priorities in critical care,* ed 3, St Louis, 2000, Mosby.

Boyer MJ: *Lippincott's need-to-know ECG facts,* Philadelphia, 1997, Lippincott.

Casey P: Management of patients with dysrhythmias and conduction problems. In Smeltzer S, Bare B, editors: *Brunner and Suddarth's textbook of medical-surgical nursing,* ed 9, Philadelphia, 2000, Lippincott.

Davenport J, Morton PG: Identifying nonischemic causes of life-threatening arrhythmias, *Am J Nurse* 97(11):50, 1997.

NCLEX® Review

1. Why would a patient have premature ventricular contractions during endotracheal suctioning?
   1 The suction catheter irritates the heart.
   2 The loss of volume causes hypovolemia.
   3 Oxygen is suctioned out, causing hypoxia.
   4 Potassium is lost during suctioning.

2. You are counseling Ms. Frost after she visits your clinic complaining of palpitations. Her ECG is normal but her Holter monitor shows premature ventricular contractions during her waking hours. Which of the following could you counsel Ms. Frost to avoid to reduce her symptoms?
   1 Cheese
   2 Milk products
   3 Nicotine
   4 Red wine

3. Mr. Landry is admitted to your telemetry unit for congestive heart failure. His laboratory results reveal the following: sodium of 140 mEq/L, potassium of 3.2 mEq/L, calcium of 10 mg/dL, and magnesium of 1.5 mEq/L. Which of these levels could be responsible for the premature ventricular contractions he is having with increasing frequency?
   1 Sodium
   2 Potassium
   3 Calcium
   4 Magnesium

4. Mr. Yodlowski is experiencing ventricular bigeminy and low blood pressure. Which of the following is the cause of the low blood pressure?
   1 Inadequate fluid intake
   2 Low potassium
   3 Lidocaine
   4 Decreased cardiac output

NCLEX® Review Answers

1. **3** Suctioning removes oxygen along with secretions. Hypoxemia causes premature ventricular contractions. The suction catheter does not come in contact with the heart. The small amount of secretions suctioned does not lead to hypovolemia. Potassium is not lost during suctioning.

2. **3** Nicotine stimulates the sympathetic nervous system to increase the heart rate and can cause premature ventricular contractions in a normal person. Milk, cheese, and red wine do not stimulate the sympathetic nervous system.

3. **2** Hypokalemia related to potassium is a frequent and notorious cause of premature ventricular contractions. All of Mr. Landry's other laboratory levels (sodium, magnesium, calcium) are within normal limits.

4. **4** Cardiac output is decreased because every other beat in the premature ventricular contraction represents incomplete ventricular filling; thus, blood pressure is decreased. Inadequate fluid volume can cause hypotension, but in this case it is not the problem. Low potassium can cause ventricular bigeminy but does not directly cause hypotension. Lidocaine is used to *treat* PVCs; it does not *cause* them.

Notes

Chapter 12
Practice Strips

Please analyze and identify information for each of the following ECG strips.

Strip 1   Rate: _____   Rhythm: _____   P wave: _____

          PR interval: _____   QRS: _____

          Rhythm interpretation: _____

Strip 2   Rate: _____   Rhythm: _____   P wave: _____

          PR interval: _____   QRS: _____

          Rhythm interpretation: _____

Strip 3   Rate: _____   Rhythm: _____   P wave: _____

PR interval: _____   QRS: _____

Rhythm interpretation: _____

13 Ventricular Tachycardia

What You WILL LEARN

After reading this chapter, you will know how to do the following:

✔ Define ventricular tachycardia (VT).

✔ Describe the electrocardiogram (ECG) characteristics of VT.

✔ Differentiate among treatment of stable VT, unstable VT, and pulseless VT.

What IS Ventricular Tachycardia?

Ventricular tachycardia (VT) is defined as three or more consecutive, premature ventricular contractions (PVCs) in a row, with a ventricular rate that exceeds 100 beats per minute (bpm). It can occur without warning, or it may be preceded by some sign of ventricular irritability (e.g., PVCs). It is commonly referred to as "v. tach."

What You NEED TO KNOW

Recognition

VT can last from a short run of three PVCs (sometimes called a salvo) to a sustained, continuous rhythm. The two factors that determine how well the patient tolerates the rhythm are (1) the ventricular rate and (2) the presence or absence of myocardial dysfunction, such as ischemia or infarction. The figure below shows an example of a short "run" or "burst" of VT, and an example of "sustained VT."

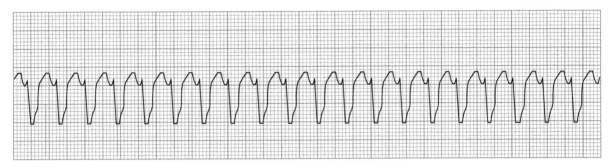

Sustained v. tach.

Redrawn from Cohn, Gilroy-Doohan: *Flip and see ECG,* Philadelphia, 1996, Saunders, p. 89.

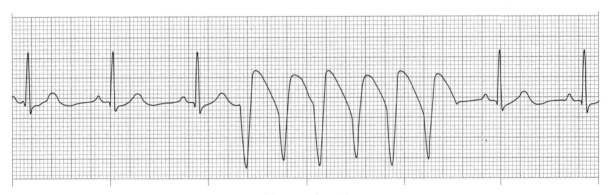

Short run of v. tach

The longer, more sustained, and the faster the rhythm, the more dangerous it is. The more rapid the heart rate, the less time the ventricles have to fill with blood between beats, and the patient's cardiac output falls. A drop in cardiac output decreases blood supply to the vital organs.

The patient may or may not have a pulse, and the tachycardia rhythm can deteriorate into ventricular fibrillation (VF) and cardiac standstill. Therefore it must be recognized and treated immediately.

 VT is one of the truly life-threatening heart rhythms.

What You NEED TO KNOW

Causes of Ventricular Tachycardia

The same conditions that cause PVCs can cause VT. VT is primarily caused by ischemia of the heart. It occurs most frequently in patients with underlying heart disease, including coronary syndrome, heart failure, and ventricular aneurysm. The most commonly encountered acute causes are ischemia, hypoxemia, hypokalemia, and digitalis toxicity.

Reperfusion after thrombolytic therapy is another cause of VT. Any drug that stimulates the sympathetic nervous system can initiate ventricular irritability. In addition, illegal cardiac stimulants (cocaine) increase oxygen demand in the heart and can lead to VT (see Chapter 20). Cardiac drugs, such as procainamide (Pronestyl), quinidine, and amiodarone, or electrolyte disturbances can lead to prolongation of the QT interval, which can precipitate polymorphic VT.

Be vigilant of the patient with a history of vomiting and/or diarrhea who is NPO (nothing by mouth) for more than 24 hours. Dehydration and loss of potassium can cause VT.

What You DO

The characteristics of VT are very striking. There are no normal-looking QRS complexes. The sole PVC that stood out in the midst of an otherwise mundane rhythm can become a string of PVCs or a rhythm in itself.

To determine whether a rhythm is VT, you should observe for the following:

- **Rate:** Atrial rate is not usually countable. Ventricular rate is between 100 and 250 bpm.
- **Rhythm:** Ventricular rhythm is usually regular, but it can be slightly irregular.
- **P waves:** No consistent P waves associated with the QRS are evident, because the rhythm is not coming from the sinoatrial (SA) node. There may be *dissociated* P waves scattered throughout.
- **PR interval:** There are none.
- **QRS:** Complex is wide and bizarre-shaped (> 0.12 seconds).

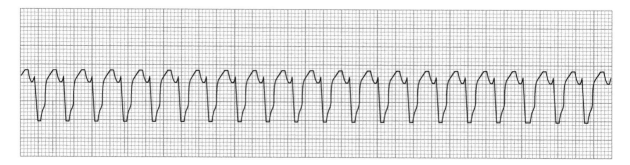

- **Monomorphic VT:** Beats arise from the same focus, and therefore all look alike
- **QT:** QT intervals are within normal limits; T wave is in the opposite direction of the QRS.

Do You UNDERSTAND?

DIRECTIONS: **Place a check by the characteristics of VT.**

1. _____ Atrial rate between 60 and 100 bpm
2. _____ Ventricular rate greater than 100 bpm
3. _____ PR interval within normal limits
4. _____ QRS between 0.06 and 0.10 seconds
5. _____ QRS greater than 0.12 seconds
6. _____ T wave opposite the normal QRS
7. _____ QT interval within normal limits
8. _____ QRS wide and bizarre

What You NEED TO KNOW

Proper treatment of monomorphic VT is totally dependent upon the effect of the dysrhythmia on the patient. According to the American Heart Association's *Advanced Cardiac Life Support* (ACLS), the following three possible scenarios and accompanying treatment algorithms may be present:
1. The patient has a pulse and is stable.
2. The patient has a pulse but is hemodynamically unstable.
3. The patient has no pulse.

What You DO

The *universal algorithm* states that there are certain presumed actions taken in all patients being monitored. These include the initial assessment of the patient's airway, breathing, and circulation (ABCs), knowledge of a

Answers: 2, 5, 6, 7, 8.

brief history of the patient's reason for being there, attachment to a cardiac monitor, the presence of a patent intravenous (IV) line, and supplemental oxygen (nasal cannula or nonrebreather mask), if needed.

When working with a patient with VT, you should remember the following:

- To document and quickly assess the rhythm strip. Because of the HR and QRS shape, the monitor will most likely alarm and run a strip automatically.
- To assess the patient's hemodynamic status (i.e., pulse, blood pressure, level of consciousness) and any other symptoms (e.g., chest pain, shortness of breath).
- To prepare to treat based on the patient's symptoms.

Treatment for Stable Ventricular Tachycardia

Short runs of VT are often well tolerated and do not require treatment; however, they should be reported and documented. In some patients, even sustained VT may not cause symptoms—at least for short periods of time. The treatment of VT depends on how the rhythm affects the patient. If the patient has an adequate pulse and blood pressure and is alert and talking with no symptoms of chest pain, shortness of breath, or dizziness, he or she is considered stable.

Sustained VT in a stable patient is treated with oxygen and medication. Drugs of choice include either lidocaine or amiodarone. Lidocaine is usually given 0.50 to 0.75 mg/kg as an IV bolus (pushed from the syringe straight into the IV line). If the VT resolves, an IV drip is hung (1 g in 250 mL) at 2 to 4 mg/min to maintain a therapeutic drug level.

Amiodarone 150 mg IV is given over 10 minutes initially. Then another 360 mg is given over the next 6 hours, and a maintenance infusion of 540 mg over the next 18 hours.

If the VT does not resolve, procainamide is the recommended second-line agent. Procainamide takes longer to work and has a greater potential for lowering blood pressure. Given as a steady infusion at 20 to 30 mg/min, the end points of procainamide administration are hypotension, a maximum of 17 mg/kg, greater than 50% widening of the QRS, or termination of the VT. In other words, administration of procainamide will cause the VT rhythm to disappear or the patient's condition will worsen and threaten life. The drug should be administered until the patient either gets better or worse.

Treatment for Unstable Ventricular Tachycardia

If the patient has a pulse but is exhibiting chest pain, hypotension, decreased level of consciousness, shortness of breath, or pulmonary edema, the VT is considered unstable. These symptoms are caused by decreased tissue perfusion secondary to decreased cardiac output, because the ventricles are beating so rapidly that there is not time for adequate ventricular filling between beats. The patient may appear pale, gray, or diaphoretic and may complain of nausea, dizziness, or palpitations.

The patient may lose consciousness because of a lack of blood supply to the brain. As long as the pulse is still palpable, the following regimen of treatment is recommended:

- If the ventricular rate is greater than 150 bpm and the patient is unstable, the clinician should prepare for immediate cardioversion. Cardioversion is seldom needed for heart rates less than 150 bpm.
- To prepare for cardioversion, ensure that the patient has a patent IV.
- Connect the patient to a cardiac monitor, pulse oximetry, and a non-invasive blood pressure monitor.
- Ensure that a cardioverter/defibrillator, intubation equipment, and a suction device are available. If there is time, and the patient is alert enough to feel the shock from the cardioversion, premedication should be administered with a sedative or analgesic.
- Set the cardioverter/defibrillator to the "synchronize" mode. Ensure that the QRS is sensed.

TAKE HOME POINTS
The first-line treatment for stable VT is to administer lidocaine or amiodarone.

Chest pain, hypotension, decreased level of consciousness, shortness of breath, and pulmonary edema are symptoms of unstable VT.

TAKE HOME POINTS

Usually, the faster the rate, the more decreased the cardiac output, and the greater the symptoms.

V_1

Redrawn from Paul, Hebra: *The nurse's guide to cardiac rhythm interpretation,* Philadelphia, 1998, Saunders, p. 163.

TAKE HOME POINTS

Unstable VT is treated immediately with cardioversion. Pulseless VT must be treated immediately with defibrillation.

Synchronized cardioversion is performed beginning at 100 joules. The shock is synchronized to avoid inadvertent striking of the shock on the T wave (**relative refractory period**), which could precipitate VF.

- If the first shock is unsuccessful, the cardioverter and defibrillator should be reset on "synchronize," and the charge should be increased to 200 joules. This process can continue with the next consecutive precordial shocks delivered at 300 joules and 360 joules, respectively.

- A brief trial of medications may be given as long as it does not cause a delay in preparing for cardioversion. Lidocaine 1.0 to 1.5 mg/kg IV push may be administered by one member of the resuscitation team while another prepares the defibrillator. Second-line drugs may include amiodarone, magnesium sulfate, procainamide, and propranolol.

Treatment for Pulseless Ventricular Tachycardia

If at any time during cardioversion the patient becomes pulseless (either VT or VF), do not synchronize the precordial shock; unsynchronized defibrillation is indicated. If the patient continues in sustained VT, this is likely to lead to VF and asystole. Defibrillation is the only definitive treatment and must be instituted immediately. (See chapter on ventricular fibrillation for details.)

TAKE HOME POINTS

VT and awake, drugs they must take.

What You NEED TO KNOW

Polymorphic Ventricular Tachycardia

Polymorphic VT (PMVT) is a variation of monomorphic VT in which there is more than one focus of irritability and therefore more than one shape of ventricular beat. The focus "wanders" and causes a "spindle-shaped" rhythm with some positive and negative complexes.

PMVT can be inherited or can result from the administration of drugs (e.g., amiodarone, procainamide, ibutilide, antihistamines), which prolongs the QT interval. It is often not recognized until an acute episode occurs. This may be during a period of physical exertion such as running or playing sports.

PMVT is also known as torsades de pointes, which is French for "twisting of the points," as the tachycardia seems to twist around the isoelectric line in different directions.

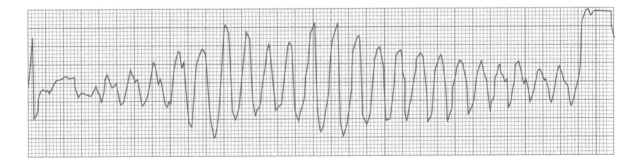

Treatment for Stable Polymorphic Ventricular Tachycardia

Treatment for stable PMVT with a prolonged QT interval is to correct abnormal electrolytes and administer magnesium or overdrive pacing. The patient's medication list should be reviewed, and any drug known to cause a prolonged QT interval should be discontinued. Alternatively, isoproterenol, phenytoin, or lidocaine can be administered to override the rate. Treatment for stable PMVT with normal QT intervals is to correct electrolyte imbalances, treat ischemia, and administer medications (e.g., β-blockers, lidocaine, amiodarone, procainamide). If these treatments fail and the patient becomes unstable, cardioversion is recommended. To prevent future episodes, it may become necessary to insert an implantable cardioverter/defibrillator.

What You NEED TO KNOW

Differentiating VT from SVT

VT is defined as a wide QRS tachycardia. It must be differentiated from supraventricular tachycardia (SVT), which is a narrow QRS tachycardia. Medical treatment differs based on the origin of the tachycardia. At times, it may be difficult to distinguish between VT and SVT. If the patient has a pre-existing ventricular conduction delay (BBB), the QRS may already be wide. Then, when the heart rate increases, although the rhythm originates above the ventricles, the QRS will still be wide. This is called SVT with aberrant conduction, and it looks like VT.

What You DO

Do not confuse SVT with VT. In general, SVT is a narrow QRS tachycardia. Because beats may be aberrantly conducted, it is often difficult to distinguish unless there is knowledge of the patient's pre-existing rhythm. It has been speculated that clinical criteria can help differentiate VT from SVT and that a patient with VT is more unstable than a patient with SVT. This premise has been disproved; some patients with VT may be more stable than those with SVT.

ECG criteria (especially QRS morphology in certain leads) are techniques that have been used to differentiate SVT with aberrant conduction from VT. This analysis may be a clinically useful strategy in the stable patient.

Because a wide QRS tachycardia of ventricular origin can be life-threatening, it is recommended that time is not wasted trying to decipher whether the rhythm is ventricular or supraventricular. Because VT is more life-threatening and less harm can be done by erroneously treating the rhythm as ventricular than by erroneously treating it as supraventricular, lidocaine is recommended as the first-line drug when there is any question about the origin of the rhythm. However, if the patient with a wide QRS tachycardia is unstable, cardioversion is the treatment of choice, regardless of the origin of the tachycardia.

Do You UNDERSTAND?

DIRECTIONS: **On the crossword puzzle below, provide the types of treatment for VT with its characteristics *(across)*. What is the treatment for unstable VT *(down)*?**

1. Second-line drug for stable VT
2. First-line alternative to lidocaine in stable VT
3. A drug for stable VT
4. Can be lethal if given in VT
5. Treatment of choice for pulseless VT
6. Helps maintain O_2 saturation greater than 92%
7. What is the treatment of choice for pulseless VT?

- Severe hypotension may lead to the development of VF.
- Administration of verapamil, a drug used to treat narrow QRS complex tachycardia, can be a lethal error in the treatment of VT, especially if the patient has atrial fibrillation with Wolff-Parkinson-White (WPW) syndrome. Severe hypotension may result, and it may lead to the development of VF.

TAKE HOME POINTS

- It is important to differentiate wide QRS tachycardia from narrow QRS tachycardia.
- If it is difficult to differentiate between VT and SVT with aberrant conduction, it should be treated as VT until proven otherwise.

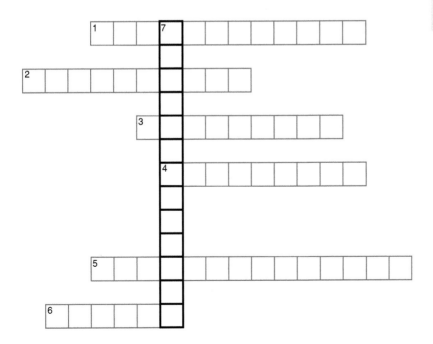

Answers: 1. procainamide; 2. amiodarone; 3. lidocaine; 4. verapamil; 5. defibrillation; 6. oxygen; 7. cardioversion.

References

Aehlert B: *ECGs made easy,* ed 2, St Louis, 2002, Mosby.

Albert CT: Common supraventricular tachycardias: mechanisms and management, *AACN Clinical Issue* 12(1):100, 2001.

American Heart Association: *Advanced cardiac life support provider manual,* Dallas, 2001, American Heart Association.

Boyer MJ: *Lippincott's need-to-know ECG facts,* Philadelphia, 1997, Lippincott.

Davenport J, Morton PG: Identifying nonischemic causes of life-threatening arrhythmias, *Am J Nurse* 97(11):50, 1997.

Hartshorn JC, Sole ML, Lamborn ML: *Introduction to critical care nursing,* ed 3, Philadelphia, 2001, Saunders.

Hazinski MF, Cummins RO, Field JM: *2000 handbook of emergency cardiovascular care,* Dallas, 2000, American Heart Association.

Huff J: *ECG workout: exercises in arrhythmia interpretation,* ed 3, Philadelphia, 1997, Lippincott.

Lewis KM: *Sensible ECG analysis,* Albany, NY, 2000, Delmar Publishing.

McCoy C: Nursing care of the patient with cardiac disorders. In Monahan FD, Neighbors M, editors: *Medical-surgical nursing: foundations for clinical practice,* ed 2, Philadelphia, 1998, Saunders.

Owen A: How to distinguish wide-complex tachycardias. Available online at www.springnet.com/criticalcare.

Paul S, Hebra J: *The nurse's guide to cardiac rhythm interpretation: implications for patient care,* Philadelphia, 1998, Saunders.

NCLEX® Review

1. Ventricular tachycardia is defined as:
   1 Atrial rate above 100 bpm
   2 Atrial rate between 90 and 160 bpm
   3 Ventricular rhythm between 100 and 250 bpm
   4 Sinus tachycardia with a ventricular rate greater than 150 bpm

2. According to Advanced Cardiac Life Support protocols, a first-line drug for stable VT is:
   1 Adenosine
   2 Lidocaine
   3 Atropine
   4 Pronestyl

3. According to Advanced Cardiac Life Support, the proper treatment for VT depends upon which of the following?
   1 Shape of the QRS
   2 Rate
   3 Age of the patient
   4 Whether the patient has a pulse or is clinically unstable

4. Mrs. Murphy is in VT at 180 bpm. She is complaining of lightheadedness and shortness of breath. Her blood pressure is 80/60. What action needs to be taken?
   1 Immediately defibrillate at 200 joules.
   2 Administer verapamil 15 mg IV push.
   3 Immediately cardiovert at 100 joules after considering sedation.
   4 Obtain a 12-lead ECG to differentiate VT from SVT.

5. First-line treatment for VT with no pulse is
   1 Defibrillation at 200 joules
   2 Synchronized cardioversion at 50 joules
   3 Lidocaine 1 mg/kg IV push
   4 Bretylium 5 mg/kg IV push

NCLEX® Review Answers

1. 3 Ventricular tachycardia originates in the ventricles and is therefore a ventricular rhythm. The atrial rate is not significant. Sinus tachycardia is not the same as ventricular tachycardia.

2. 2 Lidocaine is a drug of choice to control irritable foci in the ventricle. Adenosine is indicated in supraventricular, not ventricular, rhythms. Atropine is administered to increase the heart rate in bradycardia. Pronestyl would be given next if lidocaine is ineffective.

3. 4 Advanced Cardiac Life Support protocols recommend assessing the clinical effects of the tachycardia on the patient and then using the appropriate algorithm for stable ventricular tachycardia, unstable ventricular tachycardia, or pulseless ventricular tachycardia. The shape of the QRS, the rate, and the patient's age are not factors in treatment.

4. 3 If the patient is exhibiting chest pain, hypotension, decreased level of consciousness, shortness of breath, or pulmonary edema, the ventricular tachycardia is considered unstable. This patient is in unstable ventricular tachycardia, which requires immediate synchronized cardioversion. Defibrillation is not indicated because she has a pulse and is awake. Verapamil is not indicated; it is used for supraventricular tachycardia and can lower the blood pressure. Because the patient is unstable, time should not be wasted attempting to differentiate the source of the tachycardia by doing a 12-lead ECG.

5. 1 Defibrillation is the treatment of choice for ventricular tachycardia with no pulse. In pulseless ventricular tachycardia, it would not be effective to give lidocaine or bretylium or to perform synchronized cardioversion.

Chapter 13
Practice Strips

Please analyze and identify information for each of the following ECG strips.

Strip 1   Rate: _____   Rhythm: _____ P wave: _____

PR interval: _____   QRS: _____

Rhythm interpretation: _____

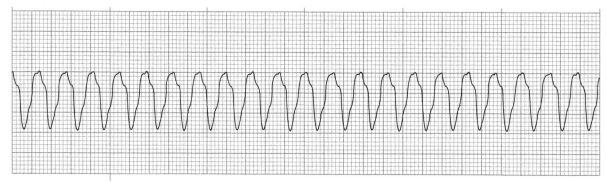

Strip 2   Rate: _____ Rhythm: _____ P wave: _____

PR interval: _____ QRS: _____

Rhythm interpretation: _____

Ventricular Fibrillation

What You WILL LEARN

After reading this chapter, you will know how to do the following:
- ✔ Define ventricular fibrillation.
- ✔ Describe the ECG characteristics of ventricular fibrillation.
- ✔ Describe the emergency treatment of ventricular fibrillation.

What IS Ventricular Fibrillation?

Ventricular fibrillation (VF) is the most frequent initial rhythm in sudden cardiac arrest. It is the single most important rhythm to recognize, because it is lethal and because it can be quickly reversed if a defibrillator is immediately available. VF is often called "v. fib."

In VF, multiple areas within the ventricles fire at random, asynchronous times, which produces a chaotic, completely disorganized rhythm, almost like a *seizure* of the heart. There is no effective contraction; the ventricles just quiver and twitch. As a result, there is no cardiac output, no pulse, and no blood pressure (BP). The patient is clinically dead and will become biologically dead unless the rhythm is swiftly terminated.

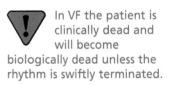 In VF the patient is clinically dead and will become biologically dead unless the rhythm is swiftly terminated.

What You NEED TO KNOW

The VF rhythm has no countable atrial or ventricular rate.

The electrical activity on the ECG monitor is composed of coarse electrical waveforms that vary in size and shape. There are no measurable intervals; consequently the PR, QRS, and QT intervals are unobtainable. This rhythm is without pattern, and all of the normal characteristics are absent. VF rhythm may be mistaken for artifact at first glance.

Redrawn from Cohn, Gilroy-Doohan: *Flip and see ECG*, Philadelphia, 1996, Saunders, p. 91.

The VF rhythm on an ECG has these characteristics:
- **Rate:** Unobtainable and too fast to count (rapidly undulating waveforms)
- **Rhythm:** Grossly irregular
- **PR interval:** Unobtainable; absent P waves
- **QRS:** Unobtainable
- **QT:** Unobtainable

Patients who suddenly display VF rhythm often have significant heart disease. Many have had a history of myocardial infarction or heart failure. Patients at high risk for recurrent VF may have surgically implanted automatic implantable cardioverter defibrillators (AICDs).

Causes of VF

Ventricular tachycardia (VT) may deteriorate into VF within minutes if not terminated. VF may also be caused by a strong stimulus at the wrong time in the vulnerable period of the cardiac cycle (i.e., middle of the T wave) or if the patient is inadvertently shocked at this point.

The same medications that cause premature ventricular contractions (PVCs) and VT can lead to VF. Hypoxia, acidosis, and electrolyte imbalances can also cause VF. In addition, VF can develop from electrical shock (e.g., shock from lightening strike or electrical devices). Because there is no pulse with VF, death will occur within 4 to 6 minutes if the patient is not defibrillated. In the hospital setting, defibrillators must be present on every nursing unit. The American Heart Association has also supported a campaign to make automatic external defibrillators (AEDs) available in nonmedical public places, such as airports and convention centers. AEDs sense the presence of VF and shock the patient only if indicated. They are intended for use by nonmedical personnel and require minimal training to use.

What You DO

When recognizing a VF pattern on a monitor, you should remember the following:

- To assess the patient's airway, breathing, and circulation (ABCs) quickly to rule out artifact (e.g., a loose electrode or movement) as the cause of the VF pattern. The patient with VF will be unresponsive, will have no pulse, and will not be breathing. There may also be accompanying seizures due to cerebral hypoxia.
- To administer cardiopulmonary resuscitation (CPR) in a pulseless patient only until the defibrillator is available. Electrical defibrillation is the definitive treatment for VF. A defibrillator must be obtained immediately.
- To never delay defibrillation while waiting for drugs, intravenous access, intubation, or CPR.
- To immediately defibrillate the patient. This step is the top priority.
- Place gelled paddles or hands-free electrodes over the right upper sternal border and apex. Ensure that the defibrillator is in the "defibrillate" mode, not the "synch" or "synchronized" mode.

 Never delay defibrillation while waiting for drugs, intravenous intubation, or CPR.

TAKE HOME POINTS

Defibrillation is an electrical charge applied externally to the heart from paddles or large electrode pads that are placed firmly on the chest. When discharged, a strong electrical shock fires all cardiac cells of the heart at one time. The cycle of the fibrillating heart must be broken so that the sinoatrial (SA) node may again take over as the normal pacemaker of the heart. The **only** effective treatment for VF is defibrillation. The probability of successful defibrillation diminishes rapidly over time. VF tends to convert to asystole within a few minutes.

- Initially, a 200-joule (J) charge is delivered to the precordial surface. If this does not convert the rhythm, the charge is immediately increased to 300 J. If this charge still does not convert the rhythm, the charge is again immediately increased to the maximal power of 360 J.

- If these first three shocks fail to convert the rhythm, CPR is begun, and the patient is then intubated, an intravenous (IV) line is started, and a series of medications are given.

- Adrenaline (epinephrine) is the first-line drug used to "jump start" the heart. Epinephrine is a pure catecholamine, which initiates the fight-or-flight response that causes the heart to beat faster and increases blood flow to the vital organs, especially to the brain. Epinephrine 1 mg IV push may be repeated every 3 to 5 minutes with no upper limit or maximal dosage.

- The American Heart Association's Advanced Cardiac Life Support (ACLS) guidelines suggest that vasopressin 40 units (U) IV push may be given as a single dose to replace epinephrine.

- Defibrillation at 360 J is then repeated. If VF is still present, a series of drugs should follow: amiodarone or lidocaine, then magnesium, and finally procainamide.

- The antidysrhythmic drugs are alternated with successive defibrillations at 360 J until the VF resolves. The goal is for the drug to help increase the fibrillation threshold, and the goal of the shock to break the cycle of the fibrillation. The sequence is drug-shock-drug-shock.

- If there is known preexisting metabolic acidosis, sodium bicarbonate may be administered to help the heart respond to the shock. In addition, as minutes go by and the heart becomes more hypoxic and acidotic, coarse VF will become finer and less likely to respond to defibrillation. Oxygen and epinephrine help make fine VF coarser so that it will more likely respond to the shock.

TAKE HOME POINTS

The order of drugs given in VF is as follows:
- Epinephrine
- Amiodarone or lidocaine
- Magnesium
- Pronestyl

Fine v. fib

- If an IV cannot be obtained, emergency drugs may be administered with endotracheal (ET) intubation. Narcan (naloxone), atropine, Valium (diazepam), epinephrine, and lidocaine (NAVEL) can all be administered by this route. The dose is doubled and is squirted down the ET tube followed by 10 mL normal saline and dispersed by manually ventilating the patient. Lidocaine and epinephrine are indicated in VF. Valium is not indicated in a cardiac arrest situation. Atropine is used in asystole and bradycardia, and Narcan is used to reverse narcotic overdose.
- Secondary assessment is now indicated for ABCs: Airway (ET tube, laryngeal mask airway, or Combi tube), Breathing (assess by an end-tidal carbon dioxide monitor), and Circulation (monitor pulse and BP, and secure IV access). NOTE: If the pulse is not present, there can be no BP present.

TAKE HOME POINTS

Traditional defibrillation uses a monophasic waveform, in which current flows between the electrodes on the chest in one direction only. With the newer biphasic defibrillation, electrical current flows in one direction, then reverses and flows back the other way. Some studies show that there is greater first shock success and less myocardial damage with biphasic defibrillation. The optimal energy level for biphasic defibrillation has not yet been determined, although less voltage may be required than with traditional monophasic defibrillation.

Do You UNDERSTAND?

DIRECTIONS: **Fill in the blanks.**

1. Name four characteristics of VF.

   _____

   _____

   _____

   _____

DIRECTIONS: **Indicate in the spaces provided whether the following statements are *true* or *false*.**

2. _____ Lightning can cause VF.
3. _____ The PR interval in VF is greater than 0.12 seconds.
4. _____ During VF the patient is biologically dead.
5. _____ Hypokalemia, hypomagnesemia, and hypocalcemia can cause VF.
6. _____ VF is associated with sudden cardiac death.

Answers: 1. **No P waves, no QRSs, no rates to count, no regular rhythm, chaotic and disorganized, no conduction intervals to count;** 2. true; 3. false; 4. false; 5. true; 6. true.

DIRECTIONS: **Fill in the blanks.**

7. Emergency stopping of all heart activity with an unsynchronized electrical charge is called _____.

8. The correct amount of joules for the initial three shocks in VF is _____, _____, and _____,

9. _____ "jump starts" the heart and helps convert a fine VF to a coarse VF, which is more likely to respond to the shock.

10. The order of drugs administered during VF might include the following:

    _____,

    _____,

    _____,

    _____,

    and _____.

11. _____ _____

    is given in metabolic acidosis (either known preexisting or confirmed by arterial blood gases).

12. A type of defibrillation in which the energy travels in one direction and then turns around and travels back in the opposite direction is called _____.

References

Aehlert B: *ECGs made easy,* ed 2, St Louis, 2002, Mosby.

American Heart Association: *Advanced cardiac life support provider manual,* Dallas, 2001, American Heart Association.

Banasik J: Heart failure and dysrhythmias: common sequelae of cardiac diseases. In Copstead LC, Banasik J, editors: *Pathophysiology: biological and behavioral perspectives,* ed 2, Philadelphia, 2000, Saunders.

Boyer MJ: *Lippincott's need-to-know ECG facts,* Philadelphia, 1997, Lippincott.

Cohn EG, Gilroy-Doohan M: *Flip and see ECG,* Philadelphia, 1995, Saunders.

Davenport J, Morton, PG: Identifying nonischemic causes of life-threatening arrhythmia's, *Am J Nurs* 97(11):50, 1997.

Hartshorn JC, Sole ML, Lamborn ML: *Introduction to critical care nursing,* ed 3, Philadelphia, 2001, Saunders.

Huff J: *ECG workout: exercises in arrhythmia interpretation,* ed 3, Philadelphia, 1997, Lippincott.

Lewis KM: *Sensible ECG analysis,* Albany, NY, 2000, Delmar Publishing.

McCoy C: Nursing care of the patient with cardiac disorders. In Monahan FD, Neighbors M, editors: *Medical-surgical nursing: foundations for clinical practice,* ed 2, Philadelphia, 1998, Saunders.

Owen A: *How to distinguish wide-complex tachycardias.* Available online at www.springnet.com/criticalcare.

Paul S, Hebra J: *The nurse's guide to cardiac rhythm interpretation: implications for patient care,* Philadelphia, 1998, Saunders.

NCLEX® Review

1. Jamie Funk is a student working in your telemetry unit and taking care of Mr. Johns, who has been known to go into ventricular fibrillation. Jamie wants to be prepared to help with Mr. Johns. You know she understands the concept of defibrillation when she states:
   1 "We will be using a small amount of energy to shock his heart."
   2 "We must set the machine up to avoid the R wave and fire on the T."
   3 "We will give Mr. Johns sedation before shocking him."
   4 "Up to three consecutive shocks (at energy settings of 200, 300, and 360) may need to be delivered."

2. Which of the following describes ventricular fibrillation:
   1 Countable
   2 Regular
   3 Synchronous
   4 Chaotic

3. Ventricular fibrillation may be preceded by:
   1 Ventricular tachycardia
   2 Pericarditis
   3 Tuberculosis
   4 Complete heart block

4. Mr. Maiorino has been brought into the emergency department with hypoxia, acidosis, and severe electrolyte imbalances. His cardiac status is of utmost concern to you because:
   1 These are causes of ventricular fibrillation, which can lead to cardiac arrest.
   2 Hypoxia can lead to further lung failure.
   3 Acidosis causes cardiac necrosis.
   4 Electrolyte imbalances cause pericarditis, which can lead to cardiac dysrhythmias.

5. Lidocaine, Atropine, Narcan, and Epinephrine (LANE) may be given by what route to an intubated patient with no IV access?
   1 Oral
   2 Down the endotracheal tube
   3 Subcutaneous
   4 Intrathecally into the spinal cord

NCLEX® Review Answers

1. 4 In defibrillation, a 200-joule charge is initially delivered to the precordial surface. If this does not convert the ventricular fibrillation rhythm, the charge is increased to 300 joules. If this still does not convert the rhythm, the charge is increased to the maximal power of 360 joules. Defibrillation delivers a strong electrical charge to the heart, firing all cardiac cells at once. Setting up the machine to avoid firing on the T wave refers to cardioversion. The patient will be unconscious and therefore not need sedation before defibrillation.

2. 4 There is no regular pattern or synchrony to the ventricular fibrillation rhythm, which therefore is chaotic. Ventricular fibrillation is not countable as there are no P waves or QRS complexes. Ventricular fibrillation is irregular because of the quivering ventricles.

3. 1 An untreated ventricular tachycardia may lead to ventricular fibrillation. Pericarditis is an inflammation of the pericardium, which is usually not life threatening unless it develops into cardiac tamponade. Tuberculosis may lead to hemorrhage but not to ventricular fibrillation in and of itself. Complete heart block may lead to asystole but not ventricular fibrillation.

4. **1** Ventricular fibrillation has electrolyte disturbances, hypoxia, and acidosis as risk factors and
can lead to cardiac arrest.

5. **2** Lidocaine, atropine, Narcan, and epinephrine
medications may be administered down the
endotracheal tube so that they can reach the alve-
oli blood supply quickly. The acronym NAVEL
may also be used (narcan, atropine, valium,
epinephrine, lidocaine).

Chapter 14
Practice Strips

Please analyze and identify information for each of the following ECG strips.

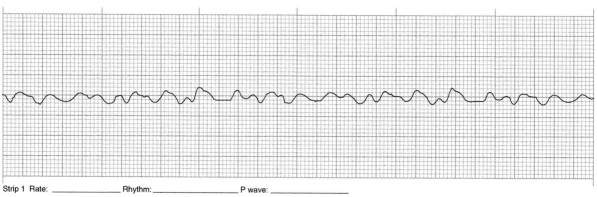

Strip 1 Rate: _____ Rhythm: _____ P wave: _____

PR interval: _____ QRS: _____

Rhythm interpretation: _____

Strip 2 Rate: _____ Rhythm: _____ P wave: _____

PR interval: _____ QRS: _____

Rhythm interpretation: _____

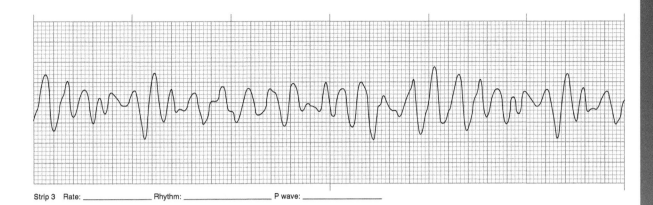

Strip 3   Rate: _____   Rhythm: _____   P wave: _____

PR interval: _____   QRS: _____

Rhythm interpretation: _____

Chapter

15

Introduction to Idioventricular Rhythms

What You WILL LEARN

After reading this chapter, you will know how to do the following:

✔ Define idioventricular (ventricular escape) rhythm (IVR).
✔ List two patient conditions in which IVR can occur.

TAKE HOME POINTS

Do not mistake IVR for PVC in interpretation of the electrocardiogram (ECG) strip.

Wide QRS complex rhythms may arise as a backup or escape rhythm if higher pacemakers fail as seen in **idioventricular rhythm**. Wide complex rhythms may also arise as an ectopic occurrence when an irritable ventricular focus fires at an accelerated rate faster than higher pacemakers, thereby taking over as pacemaker, as seen in **ventricular tachycardia**. In this chapter, idioventricular rhythms, which are escape rhythms, are discussed. Ventricular tachycardia is an ectopic rhythm discussed in Chapter 13.

What IS Idioventricular (Ventricular Escape) Rhythm?

Idioventricular rhythm (IVR) is an **escape rhythm**, which means that it occurs when both higher pacemakers, the SA node, and the AV node, either fail to initiate an electrical impulse and deliver it to the ventricles or significantly slow the rate of conduction to the ventricles. The ventricles themselves, not receiving an electrical impulse, initiate their own pacing impulse to maintain a heartbeat for survival; thus, *escaping* death.

Not receiving an electrical impulse, a site in either the bundle branches or the Purkinje fibers in one of the ventricles will take over as pacemaker and pace the heart at an inherent rate of 20 to 40 beats per minute (bpm). Idioventricular rhythm is regular, P-wave is absent, QRS is ≥ 0.12 seconds, and the T-wave is inverted due to abnormal repolarization.

Sometimes IVR may increase in rate from 20 to 40 bpm, to 41 to 100 bpm. This is called **accelerated idioventricular rhythm** (AIVR). AIVR is a ventricular arrhythmia with a gradual onset. Its appearance is exactly like IVR, except the rate is 41 to 100 bpm.

AIVR occurs most commonly due to enhanced automaticity of a ventricular pacemaker, which occurs with successful reperfusion after thrombolytic therapy for myocardial infarction.

AIVR is fairly benign, short lasting, with a good prognosis. It usually requires no therapy, and resolves as the SA node accelerates to a rate greater than the ventricular pacing site. AIVR can also occur from myocardial ischemia (especially inferior wall ischemia), digoxin toxicity, electrolyte imbalance (e.g., hypokalemia), hypoxemia, and following myocardial infarction.

What You NEED TO KNOW

IVR is a wide QRS complex escape rhythm to protect life when higher pacemakers fail. Escape rhythms are rhythms that are initiated from pacemaker sites other than the SA node. Recall that all cardiac tissue is capable of automaticity (pacemaker activity), which is a spontaneous, self-initiation of an action potential resulting in depolarization. To avoid cardiac chaos, there are three main centers of automaticity:
1. The SA node, which has the highest or strongest level
2. The AV node, which is the next level
3. A site in the ventricles that provides the lowest level of automaticity

When the SA node fails as pacemaker, the next level pacemaker (that is, the AV node) will take over as the backup or escape pacemaker maintaining a regular rhythm initiated in the AV node. This is called AV node or junctional escape rhythm (see Chapter 11). If both the SA and AV node fail, the next level pacemaker will take over. The next level pacemaker provides a ventricular escape rhythm that is called idioventricular rhythm (IVR). Thus, escape rhythms are the only protective backup sites of automaticity. If they are called upon, it is because the higher level site has failed. Therefore escape rhythms should not be suppressed with anti-dysrhythmic medications (such as amiodarone or lidocaine). Instead, escape rhythms should be protected and possibly supported with temporary cardiac pacing.

Unlike ventricular tachycardia, which is a wide QRS complex ectopic rhythm that should be suppressed with antidysrhythmic medication, IVR is an escape rhythm, as mentioned, and must be protected or the result can be cardiac standstill/arrest. IVR with a ventricular rate of less than 20 bpm is considered to be cardiac standstill.

Since IVR is a ventricular rhythm, meaning only the ventricles are depolarized, atrial kick is lost. The patient may experience signs of decreased cardiac output, such as dizziness, confusion, hypotension, and even loss of consciousness.

AIVR provides a ventricular rate of 41 to 100 bpm. It is slower than ventricular tachycardia (VT rate is >100 bpm) and faster than IVR (20 to 40 bpm). Antidysrhythmic medications should also be avoided, as this is a backup rhythm and will gradually subside as the SA node picks up its rate.

TAKE HOME POINTS

Do NOT administer antidysrhythmic medications to patients with IVR or AIVR, as they will suppress the only remaining functional pacemaker, resulting in asystole.

What You DO

- Notify the physician, rule out ventricular tachycardia, and document the rhythm.
- Protect against the use of antidysrhythmic medications that will suppress the ventricular pacemaker activity.
- Assess the patient for signs of decreased cardiac output by assessing stroke volume and heart rate. For stroke volume, assess for increased fluid volume/hypovolemia and venous constriction/vasodilation. If the patient is stable, monitor blood pressure and apical rate closely, and document the rhythm in the chart.
- If the patients exhibit signs of hypoperfusion (confusion, dizziness, hypotension, shortening pulse pressure, loss of consciousness), anticipate placement of a temporary cardiac pacemaker and set up for same (see Chapter 22).
- Atropine may be administered in an attempt to stimulate the automaticity rate of the SA node, thereby overriding the ventricular rate and taking back the control.
- If the IVR is less than 20 bpm, and the patient is not a DNR (do not resuscitate), cardiopulmonary resuscitation (CPR) may be necessary, until temporary pacing can be initiated with effective capture.

Do You UNDERSTAND?

DIRECTIONS: Fill in the blanks.

1. What is the inherent pacing rate of the ventricles? _____ to _____ bpm.
2. If the patient is in an IVR, and hypotensive, consider treatment with _____ pacing.
3. Antidysrhythmic medication should be _____ for patients with IRV or AIVR, because asystole can result.
4. The ventricular rate in patients with AIVR is between _____ and _____ bpm.
5. AIVR can be seen in patients treated with thrombolytic therapy after a _____ infarction.

References

Hebbar AK, Hueston WJ: Management of common arrhythmias: Part II. Ventricular arrhythmias and arrhythmias in special populations, *Am Fam Physician* 65(12), 2002.

Singh VN, Sharma RK: *Accelerated idioventricular rhythm,* August 15, 2004. Available online at www.emedicine.com/med/images/18852240EKG_IVR. jpg&imgrefurl=http.

Answers: 1. 20, 40; 2. cardiac pacing; 3. avoided; 4. 41, 100; 5. myocardial.

NCLEX® Review

1. Kesha Long is a 64-year-old female in the coronary step-down unit. She was just successfully treated with thrombolytic therapy for an acute myocardial infarction. She is stable, but her ECG is showing a wide QRS complex rhythm at a rate of 65. Which of the following cardiac rhythms could Kesha be in?
   1 Accelerated idioventricular rhythm
   2 Sinus bradycardia
   3 Ventricular tachycardia
   4 Junctional escape rhythm

2. Mr. Block is in an idioventricular rhythm. He is confused and hypotensive. Which of the following actions should the registered nurse anticipate?
   1 Immediate synchronized cardioversion
   2 Administration of lidocaine
   3 Placing the patient in Trendelenburg position
   4 Temporary cardiac pacing

3. The registered nurse explains the difference between escape rhythms and ectopic rhythms when he makes which of the following statements:
   1 Ectopic rhythms are protective.
   2 Escape rhythms are protective.
   3 Ectopic rhythms will always have a wide QRS complex.
   4 Escape rhythms will always have a wide QRS complex.

NCLEX® Review Answers

1. 1 Accelerated idioventricular rhythm. A wide QRS complex is usually seen with ventricular initiated impulses. An accelerated idioventricular rhythm is initiated within the ventricles and has a rate between 41 and 100 bpm. In sinus bradycardia, the QRS complex is narrow or normal and the rate is less than 60 bpm. In ventricular tachycardia, the QRS is wide but the rate is greater than 100 bpm. A junctional escape rhythm may have a wide QRS, but the rate will be 40 to 60 bpm.

2. 4 Temporary cardiac pacing. Temporary cardiac pacing is indicated because the patient is bradycardic and symptomatic. Synchronized cardioversion may eradicate the escape pacemaker. Lidocaine will suppress the escape pacemaker, resulting in asystole.

3. 2 Escape rhythms are protective. Escape rhythms are rhythms initiated from a backup pacemaker when a higher pacemaker fails; and they are protective. Ectopic rhythms are rhythms initiated from an irritable foci.

Notes

16 Asystole and Pulseless Electrical Activity (Ventricular Standstill)

What You WILL LEARN

After reading this chapter, you will know how to do the following:
- ✔ Define ventricular standstill, or asystole.
- ✔ Define pulseless electrical activity (PEA).
- ✔ Explain under what circumstances PEA may occur.

What IS Ventricular Standstill?

Ventricular standstill is the absence of any cardiac rhythm. It is also known as asystole. Asystole is more of a confirmation of death than a rhythm to be treated. Recovery is rare unless the cause of the asystole can be quickly reversed. As with ventricular fibrillation (VF), the patient has no cardiac output, no pulse, and no blood pressure. The pupils soon dilate and may become fixed because of the absence of blood supply to brain cells.

What You NEED TO KNOW

Patients rarely go directly from sinus rhythm to asystole. The heart will usually show some gradual slowing before stopping. There may be an occasional QRS complex or irregular P wave preceding ventricular standstill, which is known as an *agonal rhythm* (the rhythm of a dying heart). Within minutes, however, as hypoxia and acidosis are imminent, the rhythm will become a flat line.

Agonal Rhythm   Ventricular Standstill

Redrawn from Ignatavicius, Workman, Mishler: *Medical-surgical nursing across the health care continuum,* ed 2, Philadelphia, 1995, Saunders, p. 852.

Because the prognosis in asystole is very poor, the goal is to prevent the conditions that can cause asystole in the first place. When asystole does occur, the goal is to identify quickly and treat the conditions that may have caused the asystole.

Redrawn from Ignatavicius, Workman, Mishler: *Medical-surgical nursing across the health care continuum,* ed 2, Philadelphia, 1995, Saunders, p. 854.

What You DO

When recognizing the pattern of asystole on the cardiac monitor, you should remember the following:

- Identify ventricular standstill:
  Rate: None (perhaps some P waves)
  Rhythm: None
  P waves: None on a consistent basis
  PR: None
  QRS: None
  QT: None
- Confirm asystole in more than one lead before treatment.
- What appears to be asystole could be fine VF that may have a chance of converting with defibrillation. A fine VF pattern continues to have some irregular twitching or deflections on the electrocardiographic (ECG) strip. In contrast, asystole is a flat baseline on the monitor, regardless of the lead.
- A straight line may also appear if there is a technical problem with the equipment. Check to see that the leads are securely attached and that the correct lead is selected on the monitor.
- Once asystole is confirmed, cardiopulmonary resuscitation (CPR) is initiated immediately. Endotracheal (ET) intubation is performed as soon as possible, and intravenous (IV) access is established (if not already present).
- The causes of asystole are assessed. The only hope of recovery in asystole is to reverse the causes. They can be remembered by the following acronym:

Hubert **H.** Hoover **HAD** asystole.

Hubert	Hypoxia
H	Hyperkalemia
Hoover	Hypokalemia
H	Hypothermia
A	Acidosis
D	Drug overdose

- A transcutaneous pacer may be applied to the precordium to provide an artificial pacing stimulus. To have any chance of capturing the myocardium, pacing must be performed early and accompanied by appropriate drug administration.

- Epinephrine 1 mg rapid IV push is the first-line drug of choice in asystole. Its action is to "jump-start" the heart and preferentially route blood to the vital organs. It may be repeated every 3 to 5 minutes.
- Atropine 1 mg IV push is the other drug used in asystole. It blocks vagal stimulation so that the sympathetic nervous system can take over and the heart rate can increase, once the epinephrine gets it started. Atropine may be administered every 3 to 5 minutes up to a total of 0.04 mg/kg.
- If all efforts to resuscitate have failed, consider termination of efforts.

TAKE HOME POINTS
Compression rate for CPR is 100 compressions per minute for adults, children, and infants, and 120 per minute for neonates.

Do You UNDERSTAND?

DIRECTIONS: **Place a checkmark by the treatment for ventricular standstill.**

1. _____ Atropine
2. _____ Epinephrine
3. _____ Defibrillation
4. _____ Cardioversion
5. _____ CPR
6. _____ Pacemaker
7. _____ Lidocaine
8. _____ Adenosine

TAKE HOME POINTS
Chances of recovery from asystole are minimal unless the cause can be reversed.

www.circ.ahajournals.org

What IS Pulseless Electrical Activity

Pulseless electrical activity (PEA) is a mechanism in which there is electrical activity observed on the heart monitor, but there is no pulse in the patient. It *appears* by looking at the monitor that the patient has a pulse, but there is none. The question is: What would make a patient have a rhythm but no pulse? The answer is that there are several causes very similar to those in asystole. PEA is therefore treated much like asystole, except a pacemaker is not indicated because the electrical stimulation of the heart is already present.

Answers: **1, 2, 5, and 6 are treatments for ventricular standstill.**

What You NEED TO KNOW

Recognition

The rhythm of PEA cannot be recognized by specific waveform criteria because the electrocardiographic (ECG) pattern can appear as any number of rhythms. The following are a few examples of how PEA may appear. What makes it PEA is that there is no pulse associated with the rhythm.

The following strip *appears* to be sinus bradycardia, but if there is no pulse, it is PEA.

The above strip *appears* to be sinus bradycardia, but if there is no pulse, it is PEA.

The following strip *appears* to be idioventricular rhythm, but if there is no pulse, it is PEA.

The above strip *appears* to be idioventricular rhythm, but if there is no pulse, it is PEA.

The following strip *appears* to be a paced rhythm, but there is no capture of the myocardium and therefore no pulse. It is also PEA.

The above strip *appears* to be a paced rhythm, but there is no capture of the myocardium and therefore no pulse, so it is also PEA.

PEA can look like any rhythm. Do not be fooled by the monitor—ALWAYS CHECK THE PATIENT. The key to recognition is that the patient is pulseless. Does this mean that you have to insert an arterial line in every patient to know whether his or her rhythm is a true rhythm or PEA? No. PEA is usually discovered in a cardiac arrest situation. However, knowing your patient's diagnosis will help ensure the timely treatment of PEA, once discovered.

What You DO

- Check ABCs.
- Initiate CPR.
- Obtain an airway and an IV.
- Administer epinephrine 1 mg IVP to "jump-start" the heart. Epinephrine may be repeated every 3 to 5 minutes.

If the heart rate on the monitor is less than 60 beats per minute (bpm), atropine 1 mg may also be given. Atropine blocks any vagal response and will let the sympathetic nervous system take over to help increase the heart rate. As in asystole, very little hope of recovery exists unless the cause is reversed. The causes of PEA and their possible treatments are listed in the following table.

TAKE HOME POINTS

The following acronym may help with the memory of the causes to consider:

For **H**ealthy **H**earts **A**nd **P**arts, **D**on't **T**reat **T**he **M**onitor, **T**reat the **P**atient!

TAKE HOME POINTS

An easy way to remember the treatment for PEA is to use the initials of the name itself:

P = possible causes
E = epinephrine
A = atropine

Hypoxia and hypovolemia are the most common causes of PEA. It is always appropriate to treat PEA with oxygen and IV fluids while assessing other possible causes.

PEA: Causes and Possible Treatments

Cause	Treatment
Hypoxia	Administer 100% oxygen
Hypovolemia	Administer fluid bolus.
Acidosis	Hyperventilate and administer sodium bicarbonate.
Potassium (too high)	Administer IV glucose, insulin, and sodium bicarbonate to drive potassium back into the cell and calcium gluconate to counteract the negative inotropic effects on the myocardium.
Potassium (too low)	Supplemental intravenous potassium—ALWAYS DILUTE—NEVER GIVE IV PUSH
Drug toxicity	Administer specific antidote.
Tension pneumothorax	Initiate chest decompression with a needle or chest tube.
Tamponade (cardiac)	Initiate needle pericardiocentesis.
Myocardial infarction	Oxygen, nitroglycerin, morphine, aspirin. Consider thrombolytics or percutaneous coronary intervention.
Temperature (too low)	Warm the patient.
Pulmonary embolus	Not immediately treatable because it is not easily recognizable. If suspected, give thrombolytic drug.

Do You UNDERSTAND?

DIRECTIONS: **Complete the crossword puzzle.**

Across

1. Inadequate oxygenation
2. Cold body temperature
5. Too much acid
6. Can be too low or too high
7. Tension _____
9. Blood clot in the lung (abbreviation)

Down

1. Not enough fluid volume
3. Drug overdose causes _____
4. Heart attack (abbreviation)
8. Blood in the pericardial sac

Answers: Across: 1. hypoxia, 2. hypothermia, 5. acidosis, 6. potassium, 7. pneumothorax, 8. PE;
Down: 1. hypovolemia, 3. toxicity, 4. MI, 8. tamponade.

References

Aehlert B: *ECGs made easy,* ed 2, St Louis, 2002, Mosby.

American Heart Association: *Advanced cardiac life support provider manual,* Dallas, 2001, American Heart Association.

Boyer MJ: *Lippincott's need-to-know ECG facts,* Philadelphia, 1997, Lippincott.

Clochesy JM et al: *Critical care nursing,* ed 2, Philadelphia, 1996, Saunders.

Davenport J, Morton PG: Identifying nonischemic causes of life-threatening arrhythmias, *Am J Nurs* 97(11):50, 1997.

Earl W: *Procedures checklists: fundamentals of nursing—concepts, process, and practice.* Aspen, CO, 2000, Saddle Ruin: Prentice Hall Health.

Hartshorn JC, Sole ML, Lamborn ML: *Introduction to critical care nursing,* ed 3, Philadelphia, 2001, Saunders.

Huff J: *ECG workout: exercises in arrhythmia interpretation,* ed 3, Philadelphia, 1997, Lippincott.

Ignatavicius DD, Workman ML, Mishler MA: *Medical-surgical nursing across the health care continuum,* Philadelphia, 1999, Saunders.

Lewis KM: *Sensible ECG analysis,* Albany, NY, 2000, Delmar Publishing.

McCoy C: Nursing care of the patient with cardiac disorders. In Monahan FD, Neighbors M, editors: *Medical-surgical nursing: foundations for clinical practice,* ed 2, Philadelphia, 1998, Saunders.

Owen A: *How to distinguish wide-complex tachycardias.* Available online at www.springnet.com/criticalcare.

Paul S, Hebra J: *The nurse's guide to cardiac rhythm interpretation: implications for patient care,* Philadelphia, 1998, Saunders.

NCLEX® Review

1. Which of the following treatments is used for asystole?
   1 Defibrillation
   2 Cardioversion
   3 Pacemaker insertion
   4 Lidocaine

2. The initial treatment for ventricular standstill is:
   1 Cardiopulmonary resuscitation
   2 Defibrillation
   3 Cardioversion
   4 Pacemaker insertion

3. All of the following rhythms may cause a patient to be pulseless except:
   1 PEA
   2 Ventricular fibrillation
   3 Asystole
   4 Premature ventricular contractions

4. While assessing causes of PEA, treatment should include CPR and:
   1 potassium supplementation
   2 insertion of a chest tube
   3 100% oxygen and fluid bolus
   4 pericardiocentesis

5. The first drug administered in cardiac standstill is:
   1 Intravenous epinephrine
   2 Intravenous digoxin
   3 Intravenous potassium
   4 Intravenous lidocaine

NCLEX® Review Answers

1. 3 Pacemakers try to stimulate the heart when there is no stimulus from the heart itself. Defibrillation treats ventricular fibrillation. Cardioversion treats tachycardia. Lidocaine is used to treat ventricular dysrhythmias.

2. 1 Cardiopulmonary resuscitation is performed because the body has no perfusion to the brain and vital organs. Defibrillation is the treatment for ventricular fibrillation. Cardioversion is the treatment for ventricular tachycardia. Pacemaker insertion comes after cardiopulmonary resuscitation because it is not as immediately available.

3. 4 Premature ventricular contractions produce a weak but palpable pulse. The other rhythms (PEA, ventricular fibrillation, and asystole) do not have an obtainable pulse.

4. 3 The two most likely causes of PEA are hypoxia and hypovolemia. These two conditions should be treated initially. Potassium supplementation, insertion of a chest tube, and pericardiocentesis are only performed once a specific cause is determined.

5. 1 Epinephrine is administered to try to quickly and efficiently restart the heart. Digoxin, as a chronotropic drug, promotes a decrease in rate because it prolongs the refractory or resting time of the atrioventricular node. Potassium is administered to correct fluid and electrolyte balance. Lidocaine is used to treat ventricular dysrhythmia.

Chapter 17

Atrioventricular Blocks

What You WILL LEARN

After reading this chapter, you will know how to do the following:

✔ Define atrioventricular (AV) block.

✔ Describe the ECG characteristics of first-degree AV block

✔ Differentiate second-degree AV block, type I, from second-degree AV block, type II.

✔ Describe the ECG characteristics of complete (third-degree) heart block.

✔ Describe the treatment of first-degree, second-degree, and third-degree AV blocks.

What IS Atrioventricular Block?

Atrioventricular (AV) *block* is defined as a delay or interruption in conduction between the atria and ventricles. It is sometimes simply called *heart block* (HB). The part of the electrocardiographic (ECG) complex most affected in heart block is the PR interval, because it represents the relationship between the atria and the ventricles.

AV block is not just one block; it is a series of blocks that represent a progression in severity. These blocks range from simple prolonging of the AV conduction time (first-degree AV block) to complete lack of electrical transmission between the atria and ventricles (third-degree AV block).

HBs may be caused by ischemia, necrosis, or fibrosis along the conduction pathway, or they may be caused by delayed AV conduction due to drugs such as digoxin, ß-blockers, and calcium channel blockers.

If the ventricular rate decreases and, thus, the blood supply to the brain and body decreases, the patient may have symptoms resulting from hypoxemia. Symptoms of hypoxemia may range from lightheadedness and dizziness to temporary loss of consciousness (syncope).

AV blocks range from first to third degree. The following is a list of the least to most severe forms of AV block:

- First-degree AV block
- Second-degree AV block, type I (Mobitz type I or Wenckebach)
- Second-degree AV block, type II (Mobitz type II)
- Third-degree AV block (complete HB)

What IS First-Degree AV Block?

A *first-degree AV block* occurs when the conduction between the atrium ← constant
and ventricle is prolonged beyond 0.2 seconds (the normal PRI is 0.12 to 0.20 seconds). Think of this as driving to work or school. You know

how long it normally takes; however, if you run into an unexpected traffic delay, it will take you longer to go the same route.

PR=0.32 sec
(Normal PR ≤ 0.20 sec)

Redrawn from Cohn, Gilroy-Doohan: *Flip and see ECG,* Philadelphia, 1996, Saunders, p. 97.

What You NEED TO KNOW

In first-degree AV block, the length of time it takes for the electrical impulse to get from the atria to the ventricles is longer than normal. Therefore the PR interval is consistently longer than normal (greater than 0.2 seconds). Everything else in the rhythm strip is normal. In fact, if you do not look closely and measure the PR interval, you may see only a normal sinus rhythm (NSR) and overlook the first-degree AV block.

A first-degree AV block can be temporary or permanent. There are several possible causes. For example, ischemia secondary to swelling could cause a temporary HB after open-heart surgery or myocardial infarction (MI). AV HBs tend to occur after injury to the right coronary artery. Digoxin (Lanoxin), even at normal therapeutic doses, can cause a prolonged PR interval (first-degree AV block). Calcium channel blockers, such as nifedipine (Procardia), and β-blockers, such as metoprolol (Lopressor), can cause HBs. If medications are thought to have caused an AV block, they may be changed or discontinued.

Age-Related Specifics

HB increases in frequency in older adults. As people age, they lose pacemaker cells. Ventricular septal defects (VSDs) in young children and the surgical procedures to correct these abnormalities can cause edema and HB.

What You DO

First-degree AV block usually does not cause symptoms, so treatment is not necessary as long as the heart rate is normal. However, this rhythm could eventually lead to a more severe, higher level of block. Therefore you should monitor the patient, review the medication record, and make sure that the prescribing health care provider is aware of the condition. It is rarely an emergency, unless it is associated with a symptomatic bradycardia.

Do You UNDERSTAND?

TAKE HOME POINTS

- **ECG criterion:** First-degree AV block
- **Atrial and ventricular rates:** Greater than 60 beats per minute (bpm) but less than 100 bpm
- **Rhythm:** Regular
- **P waves:** Present and countable
- **PR interval:** Greater than 0.2 seconds
- **QRS:** Normal (one for every P wave)
- **QT:** Normal

DIRECTIONS: **Place a check next to the characteristics of first-degree AV block.**

1. _____ Atrial rate below 60 bpm
2. _____ Irregular atrial and ventricular rhythms
3. _____ PR interval between 0.12 and 0.2 seconds
4. _____ PR interval greater than 0.2 seconds
5. _____ Wide and bizarre QRS complex
6. _____ QT interval within normal limits

Answers: 4 and 6 are characteristics of first-degree AV block.

TAKE HOME POINTS

When assessing the patient with **type I second-degree** (Wenckebach) **AV block,** you should look for the following:

- **Atrial rate:** Faster than ventricular rate.
- **PR interval:** Grows progressively longer until the P wave is not conducted. (In our example, the PR interval goes from 0.16 to 0.28 to 0.36 seconds; then a P wave sits by itself.) After the nonconducted P wave, the cycle starts again with a short PR interval, and then each consecutive PR interval progressively lengthening until a beat is dropped again.
- **Atrial rate:** Faster than ventricular rate
- **Atrial rhythm:** Regular
- **Ventricular rhythm:** Irregular at the dropped QRS
- **P waves:** Appear the same (like sinus P). Will occasionally be dropped.
- **QRS complex:** Absent after the nonconducted P wave; normal configuration after other beats
- **QT interval:** Not affected, normal

What IS Second-Degree AV Block?

Second-degree HB is a more severe type of AV block that comes in two varieties: (1) type I (may be called Mobitz I or Wenckebach) and (2) type II (may be called Mobitz II, classic, or "fixed ratio"). Although they have different characteristics, communication to the ventricles is not always complete with every beat in both types. In other words, there are more Ps than QRS complexes; some Ps are not conducted.

What You NEED TO KNOW

Type I Second-Degree Block (Mobitz I or Wenckebach)

Type I second-degree block is characterized by a PR interval that may be initially normal; however, with each successive beat, the PR interval gets longer and longer until there is a P wave that sits alone. Because this beat never makes it to the ventricles, this characteristic is often called a nonconducted P wave. The cycle after the dropped P wave starts over with a normal PR that gradually gets longer until it drops again; then the cycle repeats itself. It is like the AV node is getting tired of conducting the impulses. It takes a little longer to carry each successive beat down to the ventricles. Then, finally, it takes a break and cannot conduct at all—and therefore it drops a beat. After the break, the AV node has had a chance to rest; it is rejuvenated, and can start over again with a shorter PR interval. Type I second-degree block (Wenckebach) is not difficult to recognize, but you

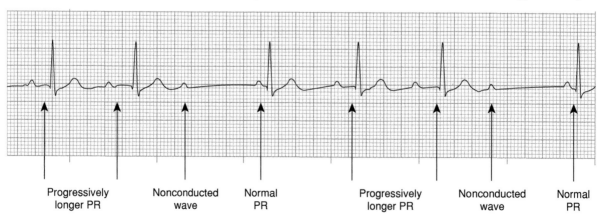

| Progressively longer PR | Nonconducted wave | Normal PR | Progressively longer PR | Nonconducted wave | Normal PR |

must be looking for it to find it. The recognition of "grouped beatings" at first glance should alert you to look for it. Wenckebach is often caused by an increase in parasympathetic tone or drug effect (digoxin, β-blockers, calcium channel blockers). It is usually transient, and its prognosis is good.

The QRS complex and QT interval are not affected because the problem is above the ventricles. Second-degree type I HB is relatively benign. It is the least serious of the second-degree blocks and rarely progresses to third-degree HB. The patient's symptoms are related to how slowly the ventricles are beating.

Type II Second-Degree Block (Mobitz II)

Type II second-degree AV block is sometimes referred to as Mobitz II, "classic," or "fixed ratio" second-degree AV block. It is more advanced and severe than Wenckebach. In type II second-degree AV block, the AV node refuses to allow certain beats through to the ventricles in a fixed ratio (every second or third beat may be dropped). The PR interval for the conducted beats remains constant.

The PR interval is what differentiates type II from type I Wenckebach. In Wenckebach, a clear warning is given by PR interval lengthening. In second-degree type II AV block, the PR interval remains constant, but the QRS complex is dropped without warning. The atrial rate may be two, three, or even four times the ventricular rate. The following example demonstrates a 2:1 block; that is, there are two P waves for every QRS complex.

> ### TAKE HOME POINTS
> When assessing the patient with **type II second-degree AV block,** you should look for the following:
> - **Rate:** Normal atrial rate; slower ventricular rate
> - **Rhythm:** Regular atrial rhythm; regular ventricular rhythm
> - **P wave:** Normal appearance. More Ps than QRSs—usually in a set pattern—i.e., 2:1, 3:1, and so forth
> - **PR interval:** May be normal or prolonged **but remains constant!**
> - **QRS complex:** Usually within normal limits; may be greater than 0.10 seconds and less than 0.12 seconds if the block is closer to the ventricles
> - **QT interval:** Duration is usually greater than 0.44 seconds

Redrawn from Ignatavicius, Workman, Mishler: *Medical-surgical nursing across the health care continuum,* ed 4, Philadelphia, 2002, Saunders, p. 680.

The rhythms of the atria and ventricles can be regular or irregular. The PR interval is consistent and usually within normal limits; it does not lengthen before a dropped beat as with Wenckebach. The QRS complexes are normal; they may be up to 0.12 seconds. The QT interval may be longer than normal because this rhythm is generally a bradycardia. Even if the patient is not symptomatic, this rhythm is dangerous because it is more likely to evolve into third-degree HB. Second-degree type II AV block is rarely the result of increased parasympathetic tone or drug effect. It is due to more serious causes, such as ischemia.

What You DO

When working with a patient with second-degree HB, you should remember the following:

1. Identify underlying causes, if possible.
2. No treatment is needed if the ventricular rate is normal and the patient does not have symptoms.
3. If the patient has symptoms such as lightheadedness or dizziness or is hypotensive, remember the following:
   - Start an intravenous (IV) line and administer atropine 0.5 to 1.0 mg intravenous push (IVP).
   - Prepare a temporary transcutaneous pacemaker, which stimulates the heart through the chest wall via electrodes attached to an external machine.
   - A temporary transvenous pacemaker may be inserted at the bedside.
   - If a permanent pacemaker is needed, it is generally inserted in the operating room or cardiac catheterization laboratory.
   - If the patient has just had open heart surgery, the temporary epicardial wires that are left in place may be connected to an external pulse generator box to pace the patient.

Do You UNDERSTAND?

DIRECTIONS: **Answer the following questions.**

1. The key feature in first-degree AV block is _____.
2. True or False: First-degree AV block is usually of no danger to the patient as long as the overall heart rate is not too slow.
3. The pattern of progressive lengthening of the PR interval until a beat is dropped is called _____.

Answers: 1. PR > 0.20 seconds; 2. True; 3. Wenckebach.

4. In classic second-degree fixed-ratio AV block (Mobitz II), what would the ventricular rate be in 2:1 block when the atrial rate is 90 bpm?

5. Which of the following are true statements about first-degree AV block? (Check each one)

_____ a. All beats are conducted through to the ventricles

_____ b. Impulses are coming from the sinoatrial (SA) node

_____ c. Ventricular conduction should be normal

_____ d. The QRS should be wide (>0.12 sec)

_____ e. Conduction through the AV node occurs faster than usual

What IS a Complete (Third-Degree) Heart Block?

A *third-degree HB,* or *complete HB* (CHB), occurs when there is no communication between the heart's atrial and ventricular conduction systems (i.e., there is complete dissociation between the two parts of the heart). The effective teamwork that makes the heart pump efficiently is gone. Although the SA node is still intact and stimulates the atria normally, the AV node cannot conduct impulses to the ventricles at all. It is like a complete roadblock. NO beats can get through.

TAKE HOME POINTS

When assessing the patient with CHB, you should look for the following:

- **Rate:** Atrial normal (60 to 100 bpm); ventricular between 20 and 40 bpm if ventricular escape; 40 to 60 bpm if nodal escape
- **Rhythm:** Regular
- **P wave:** All appear the same (sinus) in origin but not followed by a QRS. Will occur at regular intervals ("march out") unrelated to the QRS
- **PR interval:** Varying because there is no relationship
- **QRS complex:** May be normal (if nodal escape) or wide (if ventricular escape). Not related to the P waves
- **QT:** Longer than norma

CHB is the most severe form of AV block. If it were not for an escape rhythm, there would be ventricular standstill or asystole, because none of the P waves make it past the AV node to stimulate the ventricles. The underlying *escape* rhythm (the rhythm responsible for stimulating the ventricles) comes from either the AV node or the ventricles themselves.

If there is enough healthy AV node tissue, the AV node may come to the rescue. The AV node is able to initiate impulses at a rate of 40 to 60 bpm. This is slow but better than asystole. The QRS may be normal or slightly prolonged. The following is an example of CHB with a nodal escape rhythm.

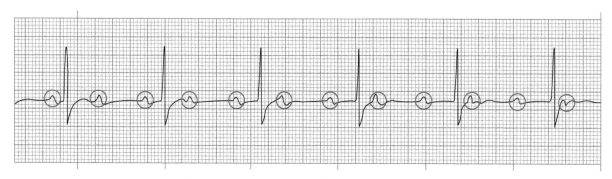

3° AVB with nodal escape rhythm. P waves are circled.

 TAKE HOME POINTS

With CHB, you will note a slow heart rate, more Ps than QRSs, and an inconsistent PR interval. The QRS rhythm will be regular and slow.

CHB with a nodal escape rhythm may be caused by increased parasympathetic tone associated with inferior MI, toxic drug effect, or damage to the AV node. This type of HB is likely to be transient and associated with a more favorable prognosis. CHB with a ventricular escape rhythm indicates the presence of extensive conductive system disease involving both bundle branches. It is more serious and more permanent, requiring a transvenous pacemaker insertion. The following example demonstrates a ventricular escape rhythm.

3° AVB with ventricular escape rhythm. P waves are circled.
Redrawn from Cohn, Gilroy-Doohan: *Flip and see ECG*, Philadelphia, 1996, Saunders, p. 103.

What You NEED TO KNOW

- In CHB, the atria beat at their own rate in a regular manner, and the ventricles do the same. However, both follow their inherent pacemaker rates, that is, the atria beat between 60 and 100 bpm and the ventricles fire at 20 to 40 bpm, if ventricular escape, or 40 to 60 bpm if nodal escape. Another way to say this is that the atria and ventricles are no longer "married" to each other. They each "do their own thing."
- The rhythm of each chamber of the heart is regular with itself (both the P-to-P interval and the R-to-R interval are regular).
- The PR intervals are inconsistent because the P waves are unrelated to the QRS complex. They are therefore not truly PR intervals.
- If the escape rhythm comes from the ventricles, the QRS complex will be wide (less than 0.12 seconds) and slow (20 to 40 bpm).
- If the escape rhythm comes from the AV node, the QRS complex may be less than 0.12 seconds, and the rate will be between 40 and 60 bpm.
- The QT interval is usually long, with a bradydysrhythmia.

 If atropine is ineffective, catecholamine infusion of dopamine or epinephrine may be started to treat CHB. A pacemaker is indicated. (Isoproterenol is rarely used because of the increased oxygen demand on the heart.)

What You DO

CHB is almost always a cause of severe symptoms in the patient because of the slow heart rate. Complaints of severe fatigue, lightheadedness, and increasing dyspnea are common. There may be a marked change in the level of consciousness. The patient may be hypotensive. These symptoms are treated similarly to type II second-degree AV block.

When working with patients with CHB, you should remember the following:
- To start an IV
- To give the patient oxygen to elevate SaO_2 levels
- To initiate transcutaneous pacing
- To prepare for insertion of a transvenous pacemaker

NOTE: Atropine is not indicated for treatment of CHB. It may increase the atrial rate but has no effect on the ventricular rate.

 TAKE HOME POINTS

If the patient is symptomatic, it is more important to treat the patient than to waste time attempting to differentiate the level of heart block.

Do not treat ventricular escape beats with lidocaine. Although they are ventricular beats, they are not premature ventricular contractions. The mechanism is different; it is the ventricles' attempt to help out a failing heart. To suppress this mechanism is to erase the only ventricular stimulation there is, and this will lead to asystole.

DO YOU UNDERSTAND?

DIRECTIONS: **Fill in the words in the crossword puzzle.**

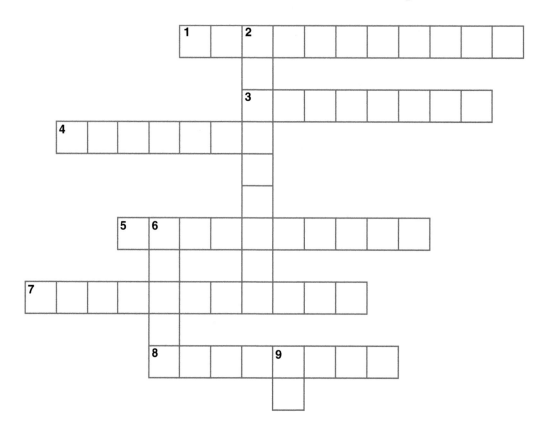

Across

1. Low blood pressure
3. Third-degree or _____ HB
4. Fainting
5. Mobitz I
7. Catecholamine infusion
8. Drug of choice in bradycardia

Down

2. Makes a spike before the QRS complex
6. Swelling
9. Interval affected in all AV blocks

References

Aehlert B: *ECGs made easy*, ed 2, St Louis, 2002, Mosby.

American Heart Association: *Advanced cardiac life support provider manual*, Dallas, 2001, American Heart Association.

Boyer MJ: *Lippincott's need-to-know ECG facts*, Philadelphia, 1997, Lippincott.

Copstead LE, Banasik J: *Pathophysiology: biological and behavioral perspectives*, ed 2, Philadelphia, 2000, Saunders.

Huff J: ECG *workout: exercises in arrhythmia interpretation*, ed 3, Philadelphia, 1997, Lippincott.

Lewis KM: *Sensible ECG analysis*, Albany, NY, 2000, Delmar Publishing.

Springhouse Corporation: *ECG interpretation made incredibly easy*, Springhouse, PA, 1997, Springhouse Corporation.

NCLEX® Review

1. Which of the following best describes a complete heart block?
   1 Prolonged PR interval
   2 Progressive prolongation of the PR with occasional dropped QRSs
   3 Every other P wave dropped
   4 Ps and QRSs each in a regular pattern but beating independently of each other

2. Mr. Brown is admitted to the progressive telemetry unit with a suspected MI. His rhythm strip indicates the development of second-degree heart block, type II. Which of the following medications would you hold until making his primary health care provider aware of the situation?
   1 Digoxin
   2 Atropine
   3 Sublingual nitroglycerin
   4 Dopamine (Intropin)

3. What is the treatment for first-degree heart block?
   1 Pacemaker
   2 Atropine
   3 No treatment unless bradycardic
   4 Defibrillation

4. All of the following symptoms may be associated with heart block except:
   1 Hypertension
   2 Syncope
   3 Decreased urinary output
   4 Confusion

5. Ventricular escape beats are treated with:
   1 Nothing
   2 Procainamide
   3 Cardioversion
   4 Lidocaine

6. In complete heart block, which part of the heart is pacing the ventricles?
   1 The SA node
   2 Either the AV node or the ventricles
   3 Either the SA node or the ventricles
   4 Either the SA node or the atria

NCLEX® Review Answers

1. 4 Complete heart block is described as Ps and QRSs in a regular pattern but beating independently of each other. Prolonged PR interval describes first-degree heart block. Progressive prolongation of the PR with occasional dropped QRSs is second-degree heart block, type I or Wenckebach. "Every other P wave dropped" is the definition for second-degree heart block, type II.

2. 1 Digoxin, as a chronotropic drug, promotes a decrease in rate because it prolongs the refractory, or resting, time of the atrioventricular node. Atropine is given for symptomatic second-degree heart block. Nitroglycerin is given for chest pain and is contraindicated in hypotension. Dopamine is given in larger intravenous doses for hypotension, which could result from second-degree heart block.

3. 3 First-degree heart block is relatively benign, and there is no specific treatment unless the heart rate drops too low; in such an instance, the treatment would be for the bradycardia, not the first-degree heart block itself. The first-degree block should be closely observed to ensure that it does not advance to a higher level. Pacemaker and atropine are only indicated in higher levels of AV block with clinical symptoms. Defibrillation is not indicated in any heart block.

4. 1 Hypotension, but not hypertension, can be a result of HB. Syncope, decreased urinary output, and confusion are symptoms that can be caused by heart block as a result of lack of oxygen to the brain and kidneys.

5. 1 Ventricular escape beats are the ventricles' attempt to help out a bad situation. If you suppress the only beats you have by administering procainamide or lidocaine or giving cardioversion, you will worsen the situation and cause asystole.

6. 2 In CHB, there is an escape rhythm either from the AV node at a rate of 40 to 60 bpm or from the ventricles at a rate of 20 to 40 bpm. The SA node is firing but cannot get past the AV node. The atria are stimulated by the P wave but are out of synchrony with the ventricles.

Notes

Chapter 17
Practice Strips

Please analyze and identify information for each of the following ECG strips.

Strip 1 Rate:_____ Rhythm: _____ P wave: _____

PR interval: _____ QRS: _____

Rhythm interpretation: _____

Strip 2 Rate: _____ Rhythm:_____ P wave: _____

PR interval:_____ QRS:_____

Rhythm interpretation:

Strip 3 Rate: _____ Rhythm: _____ P wave: _____

PR interval: _____ QRS: _____

Rhythm interpretation: _____

Strip 4 Rate: _____ Rhythm: _____ P wave: _____

PR interval: _____ QRS: _____

Rhythm interpretation: _____

Strip 5 Rate: _____ Rhythm: _____ P wave: _____

PR interval: _____ QRS: _____

Rhythm interpretation: _____

Strip 6 Rate: _____ Rhythm: _____ P wave: _____

PR interval: _____ QRS: _____

Rhythm interpretation: _____

Chapter 18

Cardiac Noninvasive Diagnostic Tests

What You WILL LEARN

After reading this chapter, you will know how to do the following:

- ✔ Explain what an ECHO (echocardiogram) is.
- ✔ List two conditions when a "Holter monitor" would be prescribed.
- ✔ Explain the purpose of a signal-averaged electrocardiogram (SAECG).
- ✔ Define what a "stress test" is.
- ✔ Name two conditions, or potential conditions, for which a stress test would be prescribed.

Several different noninvasive cardiac diagnostic tests are discussed in this chapter, including the echocardiogram (ECHO), Holter monitor, signal-averaged electrocardiogram (SAECG), and stress test.

What IS an ECHO?

A traditional transthoracic ECHO is a noninvasive acoustic-imaging procedure that examines the size and shape of the heart, as well as the position, thickness, and movement of the heart valves and chambers. An ultrasonic beam is deflected off the heart structures and received back into an oscilloscope that creates a two-dimensional (2D) image.

A transthoracic ECHO has four components:

1. **M-mode.** Provides an "ice-pick" view of the heart and a black-white and gray printout on the strip chart recorder.

2. **2D ECHO.** Provides a real-time, high-resolution view of the heart and great vessels. It can detect a pericardial effusion as little as 20 to 30 mL. Its most common use is to measure chamber size and wall thickness.

3. **Doppler echo.** Provides measurement of gradients in stenotic or regurgitant heart valves and intracardiac shunts. It also detects atherosclerosis by evaluating blood flow through the carotid arteries. Ultrasound waves are reflected off of the red blood cells (RBCs), and the frequency of these waves is altered according to the blood flow velocity. (Blood flowing through the carotid arteries produces the characteristic "swooshing" sound of each heartbeat.) When Doppler echo is combined with 2D echo, the echo may be called a duplex Doppler. *Color-flow Doppler* integrates the structural information provided by 2D echo with pulsed Doppler color-coded flow maps that depict the direction, velocity, and turbulence of blood flow through the cardiac chambers and great vessels. This information is used to estimate intracardiac pressure, valve gradients, and intracardiac shunting. It is sometimes called a noninvasive angiogram. Color-flow Doppler is particularly valuable when attempting to assess the degree of valvular dysfunction noninvasively (especially mitral regurgitation). Calculations are made through computerized instrumentation, and the studies are recorded onto a videotape or stored on digital media.

Transesophageal echocardiogram (TEE) is a special ultrasound test that uses a transmitter to generate high-frequency sound waves to take pictures of the back of the heart. Intravenous (IV) conscious sedation is given, the throat is anesthetized, and an ultrasound probe attached to a flexible gastroscope is inserted into the posterior pharynx and advanced into the esophagus. TEE shows a clear picture because the esophagus is against the back of the heart and is parallel to the aorta. This is especially useful in obese patients or patients with chronic obstructive pulmonary disease (COPD), whose transthoracic echo images are obscured by the lungs, rib cage, or both. TEE can pinpoint the site of a suspected aortic dissection, rule out the heart as a source of clots in patients who have had strokes, visualize valve defects, assess prosthetic valve function, and ensure that the left atrium is free from clots before mitral valvuloplasty is performed. Patients with atrial fibrillation of greater than 2-days duration have traditionally required several weeks of anticoagulation before and after electrical cardioversion because of the high incidence of thromboembolic events. TEE can identify whether a thrombus is present in the left atrium and therefore prevent the need for anticoagulation before cardioversion.

2D ECHO is the most common technique and is used to detect valvular problems, cardiac birth abnormalities in newborns, heart enlargement, cardiac tumor, and abnormalities in left ventricular motion. Better resolution for ECHOs occurs in children because they are thinner and the chest wall is less dense.

TAKE HOME POINTS
Three-dimensional (3D) ECHO is available in some institutions.

What You NEED TO KNOW

- A transthoracic echo can be performed at the bedside and takes about 30 to 60 minutes.
- There is no special preparation required.
- Conductive gel is placed over the third through fifth intercostal spaces to the left of the sternum, where the transducer is placed and angled.
- The patient will be asked to turn onto his or her side, with the left arm above the head to minimize the distance between the heart and the transducer (for better visualization).
- An echocardiogram is used to determine heart size, ventricular wall motion, pericardial effusion, and valve function.
- For a transesophageal echo (TEE), the patient must ingest nothing by mouth (NPO) and not smoke for several hours before the test.

What You DO

When treating patients who need a TEE, you should do the following:
- Tell them that they must lie still unless asked to move during the procedure.
- Explain that there should be no discomfort or side effects from the procedure. The patient should notify the nurse if the rare complications of hemoptysis or dyspnea occur.
- Withhold fluids and food after a TEE until the patient's swallowing and gag reflexes are restored.
- Tell the patient that a sore throat is common after the TEE procedure.

Do You UNDERSTAND?

DIRECTIONS: **Place a check mark next to the terms and statements that apply to 2D echocardiography.**

1. a. _____ Invasive test
   b. _____ Patient must be NPO
   c. _____ Conductive gel
   d. _____ Test tubes
   e. _____ Images the size of heart
   f. _____ TEE
   g. _____ Detects pericardial effusions
   h. _____ Six-dimensional picture

DIRECTIONS: **Indicate in the spaces provided whether the following statements are *true* or *false*.**

2. _____ A TEE may provide better visualization than a transthoracic ECHO in obese persons.
3. _____ ECHOs have better resolution in children than adults.
4. _____ ECHOs are useful in determining pacemaker failure.
5. _____ Frequent movement by the patient is necessary to improve resolution of an ECHO.

What IS a Holter Monitor?

A *Holter monitor* is a small, portable, electrocardiogram (ECG) recorder that the patient wears while engaging in normal activities for a specified period of time, usually 24 hours. It records every heartbeat during the time it is worn. It is commonly used to detect cardiac dysrhythmias and the ST segment and T wave changes of myocardial ischemia, and to evaluate the effectiveness of antidysrhythmic therapy. A resting ECG often does not detect these changes because the patient is lying still at the time and the heart rhythm is only monitored for a minute or so. The Holter monitor will be more likely to "catch" the dysrhythmia when it occurs because it is worn for a longer period of time during the patient's normal activities. Most systems provide at least two-lead recording, to permit

Answers: 1. c, e, f, g; 2. True 3. True 4. False 5. False.

ready differentiation of ventricular versus supraventricular dysrhythmias and easier detection of artifact.

What You NEED TO KNOW

TAKE HOME POINTS

Common symptoms of cardiac dysrhythmias are palpitations, dizziness, syncope, angina, and shortness of breath. These are also the signs of pacemaker failure.

The Holter monitor is used to record continuous electrical heart activity, usually for periods of 24 hours. It can help differentiate causes of syncope (fainting) by identifying abnormal heart rhythms. It can detect cardiac ischemia, dysrhythmias, pacemaker dysfunction, and conduction disturbances with sleep apnea syndrome. Dysrhythmias may be due to cardiomyopathy, coronary artery disease (CAD), pulmonary hypoxemia, or mitral valve disease.

The patient records all activity and symptoms experienced at all times within the 24-hour period on a small, diary-type book pad. After 24 hours, the monitor is removed. A technician will then scan the tape with a computerized scanner that will summarize significant ECG findings. The ECG from the Holter monitor is correlated to the patient's documented activity and symptoms.

Electronic Holter monitor scanners can record more than 100,000 heartbeats in a 24-hour period. Holter findings correlate with symptoms in 25% to 50% of patients tested.

Patients must keep electrodes dry and in place. Therefore they should avoid swimming and bathing during the time the Holter monitor is worn.

What You DO

AVOID
• Magnets
• Electric Blankets
• Metal Detectors
• Bathing or Swimming with Holter monitor

When treating patients who are wearing Holter monitors, you should remember the following:
• There is no special preparation for this procedure
• Three to seven electrodes are applied to skin that is free of hair (you should clip hair if necessary) and that has been cleansed with acetone. Electrodes are taped securely to minimize artifact.
• Lead placement will depend on the system used for monitoring. Commonly, modified versions of lead II (RA/LL) and lead VI (fourth intercostal space [ICS] at the right sternal border) are used so that the inferior and anterior surfaces of the heart may be monitored simultaneously.

- Check to see that the monitor has a full supply of paper (for the printed readout) and that the batteries are fully charged.
- Instruct patients to engage in normal activities and to keep a diary of when activities are performed and any symptoms that may occur.
- Explain (if appropriate) how the patient can connect the Holter monitor to the telephone to send the ECG reading over the telephone line to be printed out at the doctor's office or hospital.
- Instruct the patient when and where to return the Holter monitor.

- You should instruct patients to avoid bathing (except for sponge bath) and swimming for the time they are hooked up to the monitor, so that the electrodes remain intact.
- You should instruct patient to avoid magnets, metal detectors, and electrical blankets because they interfere with monitor recordings.

Do You UNDERSTAND?

DIRECTIONS: Connect the activities and things that a person wearing a Holter monitor should avoid. Then explain what ECG waveform results from connecting the Xs?

1. sponge
   bath
   X

   walking
   X

   electric
   blanket
   X

   apples
   X

   reading
   X

   X
   magnet

   X
   showering

   X
   eating

   X
   metal
   detector

   X
   swimming

TAKE HOME POINTS

Symptoms of dysrhythmias or pacemaker dysfunction include dizziness and syncope, palpitations, shortness of breath, or chest tightness.

DIRECTIONS: For each patient description, state a nursing intervention for a Holter monitor.

2. Hairy body

   _____

   _____

3. To wear Holter monitor for 72 hours instead of 24

   _____

   _____

4. Monitor brought back by one patient and now needed for another

   _____

   _____

Answers: 1. **magnet, showering, electric blanket, metal detector, swimming** (a P wave or a T wave results from connecting the Xs); 2. **Clip where electrodes are to be placed**; 3. **Check amount of paper on roll and replace if needed**; 4. **Replace battery.**

What IS an SAECG?

SAECG is a noninvasive ECG that is sensitive to detecting very low-amplitude, high-frequency electrical activity in the terminal QRS complex. It is similar to a regular ECG but uses computer processing to record lower level signals that do not normally appear on a standard ECG. The presence of these lower level signals suggests that certain factors (e.g., PVCs, ischemia, electrolyte abnormalities) may more easily trigger ventricular tachycardia. In SAECG, the ECG is recorded at high speed and high sensitivity. The signals are then filtered for the baseline noises that obscure late potentials from being seen on the standard 12 lead. The inability to detect low-frequency potentials in the SAECG correlates with a low risk for sustained malignant ventricular dysrhythmias. If SAECG is positive for late potentials, electrophysiologic testing is warranted because malignant dysrhythmias, such as ventricular tachycardia (VT), are likely.

The procedure takes approximately 20 minutes because the cardiac cycles are averaged over time to give an ECG reading.

TAKE HOME POINTS

- SAECG is useful in determining risk for developing life-threatening dysrhythmias in high-risk patients.
- Because the cardiac cycles are averaged over time, the test takes longer in persons who are bradycardic (less than 60 bpm) and shorter in persons who are tachycardic (greater than 100 bpm).
- SAECGs are NOT useful in atrial dysrhythmias and rhythms with wide QRS complexes (bundle branch block).

What You NEED TO KNOW

SAECG monitoring cannot be performed with a standard ECG machine unless it is specially programmed. Lead placement varies by the SAECG manufacturer, but basically, bipolar leads are placed on the anterior and posterior torso.

Ectopic beats and artifact are NOT included in the averaging of the cardiac cycles. Therefore it will take longer to complete this test in patients who have excessive ectopy or artifact.

What You DO

- There are no restrictions on food, liquids, or medications prior to this test
- Electrodes are placed on the chest in a similar manner to a standard ECG
- It is important for the patient to lie still. Make sure that the room is warm and the environment is calm to avoid restlessness or shivering. Motion artifact will result in increased testing time.

- Remove all electrical interference (i.e., put IV pumps on battery [not electricity], turn off hypothermia machines, televisions, and radios) so that artifact does not result.
- Position the patient supine or with the head of bed elevated at a 15-degree angle.
- Clip hair from potential lead placement sites; cleanse with an alcohol wipe.
- Teach patients to lie very still and try to relax their muscles during the test.

Do You UNDERSTAND?

DIRECTIONS: **Place a check next to each high-risk history that indicates a patient who will require an SAECG**

1. a. _____ Cardiac arrest
   b. _____ High blood pressure
   c. _____ Ventricular fibrillation
   d. _____ Gastrointestinal upset
   e. _____ Bradycardia
   f. _____ Bundle branch block

DIRECTIONS: **Write the nursing interventions for someone undergoing an SAECG.**

2. Electrical IV pump with fluids running

   _____

   _____

3. Electrical hypothermia blanket on

   _____

   _____

4. Patient wearing radio headphone

   _____

   _____

DIRECTIONS: **Place a check next to the requirements not necessary for someone undergoing an SAECG.**

5. a. _____ Alcohol wipe
   b. _____ Chest leads
   c. _____ Scissors or razor
   d. _____ Lying still
   e. _____ Warm, calm environment
   f. _____ Watching television

What IS a Stress Test?

A *stress test* is a noninvasive procedure that involves the monitoring of the cardiac electrical and mechanical response to continuous, progressively strenuous exercise. The exercise acts as a stress or "workload challenge" to the heart to determine its work capacity. Stress testing is used mainly to detect and evaluate the functional effects of coronary artery disease (CAD). Because physical stress causes an increase in myocardial oxygen demand, if CAD is present, this demand will exceed the supply. Ischemia will result, and characteristic ECG changes may be noted during this time. The test will also show how quickly the heart recovers after exercise.

The stress can be induced by exercise on a stationary bicycle, stair stepper, or treadmill, or it can be induced by medications (dobutamine, adenosine, dipyridamole) to increase heart rate and blood pressure. A target heart rate for the patient's age is determined. The exercise stress test identifies individuals who are prone to cardiac ischemia during activity but not at rest, and the pharmacologic stress test identifies those with known CAD or those who are unable to perform satisfactory exercise (older adults, patients with joint or respiratory problems). Patients are monitored continuously with ECG and BP measurements during a stress test.

Stress tests are often combined with myocardial perfusion imaging, which compares any specific areas of ischemia before and after exercising. Single photon emission computed tomography (SPECT) is the gold standard of myocardial perfusion imaging. The patient is taken to nuclear medicine for a baseline scan to determine perfusion at rest.

During peak exercise, a radioisotope (thallium or technetium-99m sestamibi tagged to Cardiolite) is intravenously injected, and the patient is rescanned. This test helps trace blood flow and differentiates viable myocardium from nonviable myocardium. For many patients with CAD and left ventricle dysfunction, the data obtained will determine whether the patient will benefit from coronary artery bypass grafting (CABG).

In patients who cannot walk on a treadmill, a pharmacologic agent may be used to induce an exertional state. Common drugs include dobutamine, adenosine, and dipyridamole. Dobutamine directly produces a tachycardia such as that induced by exertion. Adenosine and dipyridamole dilate the coronary arteries, increasing the blood flow to the area. This effect is similar to what happens during vigorous exercise. They are used in conjunction with a timed injection of a radioisotope. The patient is taken to Nuclear Medicine and scanned for areas of decreased perfusion and movement of the ventricular walls.

A *dobutamine stress ECHO* is an alternative to thallium imaging to evaluate coronary artery disease and ventricular wall motion in patients who are unable to exercise. Dobutamine causes an increase in myocardial oxygen demand by stimulating ß-2 receptors, which is similar to the response in exercise. Images are recorded at rest, dobutamine is given intravenously to increase the HR, and then images are re-recorded during maximal stress to the heart. Improvement of poorly moving ventricular walls at rest (in response to low-dose dobutamine) is highly predictive of viability and improvement of function.

> Adenosine should not be used in patients with known or suspected bronchoconstrictive disease such as asthma.

What You NEED TO KNOW

- During exercise, healthy coronary arteries dilate more than arteries that have blockages. Narrowed arteries cause a reduction in blood flow to the coronary arteries and decreased movement of the ventricles.
- A regular stress test takes approximately 1 hour. If nuclear imaging is performed, the test will take several hours
- Dobutamine may cause some mild side effects, which include chest tightness, dyspnea, flushing, nausea, headache, paresthesias, chills, palpitations, and anxiety. You should inform the patient that these side effects will only last a few minutes. (The half-life of dobutamine is only 2 minutes.)

Do not perform a stress test on patients with active unstable angina, ethanol intoxication, chest pain, myocarditis or pericarditis, congestive heart failure, digitalis toxicity, recent pulmonary embolism, or uncontrolled dysrhythmias.

TAKE HOME POINTS

Electrolyte imbalances and lung diseases can affect the patient's response to the stress test.

- Stress tests must be performed by health care practitioners certified in advanced cardiac life support (ACLS), exercise physiologists, physical therapists, or physicians.
- Stop the stress test if the patient develops severe chest pain, hypotension, weakness, or decreased level of consciousness or significant ECG changes.
- Adenosine should not be used in patients with known or suspected bronchoconstrictive disease such as asthma.

What You DO

- Gradually discontinue ß-blocker medications (within 72 hours if possible) before the test—per prescribing health care provider's order (see table on the following page for a list of ß-blockers).
- Instruct the patient to wear comfortable walking shoes and clothes if scheduled for exercise-induced stress test.
- Ask the patient to refrain from food, fluids, nicotine, and caffeine (tea, coffee, soda) for at least 2 to 4 hours before the test.
- In most cases, patients may take their regular medications, but you should check with the physician to see if any should be withheld.
- Explain that the patient will be asked to lie on a table with arms over the head for 20 to 25 minutes during nuclear scanning.
- Have an emergency crash cart available at all times.
- Attach appropriate ECG leads to hair-free areas and a BP cuff to the patient's arm.

ß-Blocker Medications

Generic Name	Trade Name
Acebutolol	Sectral
Atenolol	Tenormin
Betaxolol	Betoptic
Bisoprolol	Zebeta
Carvedilol	Coreg
Esmolol	Brevibloc
Labetalol	Normodyne
Metoprolol	Lopressor
Nadolol	Corgard
Penbutolol	Levatol

Continued

ß-Blocker Medications—cont'd

Generic Name	Trade Name
Propranolol	Inderal
Sotalol	Betapace
Timolol	Timoptic

NOTE: Any generic drug that ends in "olol" is a ß-blocker.

- For pharmacologic tests, ensure that the patient has a patent IV. Have appropriate medications ready, and notify appropriate personnel (cardiovascular and nuclear medicine technicians).
- For a dobutamine stress echo, establish IV access and obtain a resting echocardiogram. Then administer dobutamine by infusion pump at an initial rate of 5 to 10 μg/kg/min; double the rate every 3 minutes as ordered by the physician up to a maximum of 40 μg/kg/min. The goal is to increase the heart rate to the maximally predicted value for the patient's age. A chart will be used to determine this. The echocardiogram is repeated when the peak heart rate is reached. The patient may experience palpitations and slight shortness of breath. If the target heart rate is not reached, an intravenous bolus of atropine may be given. Labetalol may be used to reverse the tachycardia and relieve the patient's symptoms once the test is over. Nuclear Medicine is not required for this test.
- Check medication order. Remind the patient that the medication injection during the pharmacologic-induced stress test may cause temporary discomfort, but it will only last a few minutes.
- For exercise stress test, instruct patient to begin exercising.
- Run a baseline ECG.
- Terminate testing if you notice signs of ischemia (ST segment depression on the ECG of greater than 1 to 2 mm) or if maximal effort is achieved, as evidenced by dyspnea or systolic blood pressure greater than 250 mm Hg, or if the maximal heart rate for patient's age is obtained. You should also stop the test if dysrhythmias, chest pain, faintness, dizziness, or extreme fatigue occur.

Do You UNDERSTAND?

DIRECTIONS: **Select the best stress test for the following patients. Place an *E* if an exercise-induced stress test is the best or a *P* if the pharmacologic-induced stress test is indicated.**

1. _____ Patient with CAD
2. _____ Athlete's annual physical examination
3. _____ 102-year-old patient
4. _____ 56-year-old patient with "bad" knees

DIRECTIONS: **Fill in the blanks.**

5. What certification is required by a health care provider to be able to implement a stress test?

_____

6. State four types of equipment necessary for a pharmacologic-induced stress test.

_____

_____

_____

_____

DIRECTIONS: **Your patient is scheduled to have an exercise stress test in 3 hours and calls you from home to ask some questions. Place a check in the "Yes" or "No" column to indicate the answer to each question.**

	Yes	No
7. Can I take my morning potassium pill?	_____	_____
8. Can I have a cup of coffee?	_____	_____
9. Should I bring new shoes to wear on the treadmill?	_____	_____
10. Should I take my morning dose of metoprolol?	_____	_____

DIRECTIONS: **Match the following medications to their action in a pharmacologic stress test.**

11. a. Adenosine   _____ Dilates coronary arteries
     b. Dipyridamole   _____ Stimulates ß-2 receptors to directly increase HR
     c. Dobutamine   _____ Dilates coronary arteries; caution in patients with asthma

References

Adams SL et al: Ambulatory blood pressure and Holter monitor of emergency physicians before, during, and after a night shift, *Acad Emerg Med* 5(9):871, 1998.

Aehlert B: *ECGs made easy*, ed 2, St Louis, 2002, Mosby.

American Heart Association: *Advanced cardiac life support provider manual*, Dallas, 2001, American Heart Association.

Carlson MD, Thames MD: Approach to the patient with syncope. In WN Kelley: *Textbook of internal medicine*, Philadelphia, 1997, Lippincott-Raven.

Chernecky C, Berger B: *Laboratory tests and diagnostic procedures*, ed 3, Philadelphia, 2001, Saunders.

Elhendy A et al: Safety and feasibility of dobutamine-atropine stress echocardiography for the diagnosis of coronary artery disease in diabetic patients unable to perform an exercise stress test, *Diabetes Care* 21(11):1797, 1998.

Futterman LG, Lemberg L: The ECG in cardiac stress testing: a valuable, but unappreciated source of clues, *Am J Crit Care* 7(4):320, 1998.

Hill JM, Newton JL: Contrast echo: your role at the bedside, *RN* 61(10):32, 1998.

Kinney M et al: *AACN clinical reference for critical care nursing*, ed 4, St Louis, 1998, Mosby.

Koca V et al: Left ventricular thrombi detection with multiplane transesophageal echocardiography: an echocardiographic study with surgical verification, *J Heart Valve Dis* 8(1):63, 1999.

Quittan M, Cristal N, Ernst E: Exercise testing in coronary artery disease—procedures and clinical implications, *Eur J Phys Med Rehabil* 7(5):142, 1997.

Roelandt JR: Three-dimensional echocardiography: the future today, *Acta Cardiol* 53(6):323, 1998.

Sergeant LL: Tracking your outpatient's EKG with a Holter monitor, *Nursing* 16(10):47, 1986.

Yamada T et al: An approach to the detection of autonomic neuropathy by use of signal-averaged electrocardiography, *Pacing Clin Electrophysiol* 20(2):261, 1999.

Yamada T et al: Dispersion of signal-averaged P wave duration on precordial body surface in patients with paroxysmal atrial fibrillation, *Eur Heart J* 20(3):171, 1999.

Zitkus BS: Diagnostic tests: transesophageal echocardiography, *Am J Nurse* 97(9):17, 1997.

NCLEX® Review

1. An acoustic image that looks at the size and shape of the heart and heart valves is called an:
   1 Electrocardiogram
   2 Electroencephalogram
   3 Endoscopic vesselogram
   4 Echocardiogram

2. To evaluate prosthetic heart valves in an obese person, the best cardiac diagnostic test to perform would be a(n):
   1 ECG
   2 Holter monitor
   3 Transesophageal echocardiogram
   4 Signal-averaged ECG

3. Mrs. Eckroid's Holter monitor indicates pacemaker failure. What two symptoms are usually associated with this?
   1 Dizziness and syncope
   2 Diarrhea and fever
   3 Shortness of breath and leg cramps
   4 Headache and vomiting

4. A Holter monitor is commonly used to evaluate what type of drug therapy?
   1 Antihypertensive
   2 Antidiarrheal
   3 Antispasmodic
   4 Antidysrhythmic

5. The patient's apical pulse is tachycardic, and he is complaining of angina, shortness of breath, and syncope. He has a history of dizziness for the past 3 days. Based on this information, what might the patient's diagnosis be?
   1 Renal failure
   2 Cardiac dysrhythmia
   3 Brain tumor
   4 Hypertension

6. Which of the following will create artifact on the signal-averaged ECG? The patient:
   1 Is lying still
   2 Has his or her eyes open
   3 Is shivering
   4 Is lying with the head of the bed elevated 15 degrees

7. The initial dose of dobutamine for a pharmacologic stress test in an adult is:
   1 1 μg/kg/min
   2 5 to 10 μg/kg/min
   3 25 mg oral
   4 50 mg sublingual

8. You have a 42-year-old man scheduled for a stress test. Which of these factors would give you a clue that the test should be canceled?
   1 He had a pulmonary embolism 5 years ago.
   2 He had 30 mL of water this morning.
   3 He denies chest pain.
   4 He is digitalis toxic according to his blood work results.

NCLEX® Review Answers

1. 4 An echocardiogram is by definition an acoustic image of the heart and heart valves. An electrocardiogram evaluates the heart's electrical activity, while an electroencephalogram evaluates brain activity. An endoscopic vesselogram is not a real test.

2. 3 TEE evaluates prosthetic heart valves and is particularly useful in seeing the heart in obese persons. An ECG and the Holter monitor evaluate the electrical activity of the heart. A signal-averaged ECG detects low amplitude electrical activity of the heart during diastole.

3. **1** Dizziness (near syncope) is a result of a lack of steady oxygen supply to the brain. Diarrhea, fever, headache, and vomiting are not symptoms of pacemaker failure. Shortness of breath is a symptom, but leg cramps are not.

4. **4** Holter monitors monitor the heart. Antidysrhythmic drug therapy is for the heart. Antihypertensives are blood pressure medications. Antidiarrheals are to lessen stool output. Antispasmodics stop muscle spasms.

5. **2** Based on the symptoms, cardiac dysrhythmia is suspected. Renal failure, brain tumor, and hypertension would not cause angina.

6. **3** Shivering is movement, and patient movement causes artifact. The patient should be lying still. Having his or her eyes open does not affect the test. Lying with head of the bed elevated 15 degrees has no effect on detecting heart activity.

7. **2** The correct dose is 5 to 10 μg/kg/min. A dose of 1 μg/kg/min is too low to be effective. An oral dose of 25 mg is incorrect because dobutamine is only given intravenously, and 25 mg is an incorrect dose. A sublingual dose of 50 mg is also an incorrect dose and route.

8. **4** As the heart is already stressed because of too much cardiac medication, and overstressing the heart with the stress test could cause death, this patient's stress test should be canceled. Only a recent pulmonary embolism would contraindicate the stress test. Liquids need to be refrained from for 2 hours before the test. If the patient had chest pain, the stress test would be canceled, but his denial makes this unnecessary.

What You WILL LEARN

After reading this chapter, you will know how to do the following:
- ✔ Describe a 12-lead ECG.
- ✔ Define acute coronary syndrome.
- ✔ Explain in anatomic and physiologic terms a transmural infarction.

A heart attack, or myocardial infarction (MI), is the death of heart tissue. MI is usually caused by a complete blockage from a blood clot of a coronary artery narrowed by atherosclerosis. Atherosclerosis is the development of plaque from fatty-like substances that collect in the intima of the coronary artery. This narrowing of the arteries is a process that occurs over years to decades.

The area of infarction upsets the normal electrical conduction patterns and leaves a telltale electrical sign. The electrical sign from the infarction changes the electrocardiogram (ECG) dramatically.

In this chapter, the 12-lead ECG and the identification of ischemia, injury, and infarction are examined. In addition, we discuss the diagnosis of an infarction from a 12-lead ECG.

What IS a 12-Lead ECG?

The basic components of heart monitoring and the differentiation between continuous monitoring and a 12-lead ECG are discussed in Chapter 7. We examined two of the leads. In this chapter, additional leads are described.

The *12-lead ECG* examines the heart from 12 different views and provides information about what is happening in the heart. The 12-lead ECG is made up of three sections: (1) limb leads, (2) augmented leads, and (3) precordial or chest leads.

Redrawn from Copstead, Banasik: Pathophysiology, ed 2, Philadelphia, Saunders, p. 420.

What You NEED TO KNOW

Limb Leads

There are several limb leads with which you should be familiar:

- Lead I measures the current of energy from the right arm (negative pole) to the left arm (positive pole); it looks at the lateral surface of the left ventricle.
- Lead II measures the current of energy from the right arm (negative) to the left leg (positive). You should have become familiar with this lead (primary monitoring lead) in previous chapters. Lead II looks at the inferior surface of the left ventricle.
- Lead III has its negative pole at the left arm and the positive pole at the right leg. This lead (along with leads II and aV_F) looks at the inferior surface of the left ventricle. Think of the positive pole as a smiling, clever lovebird that is looking at events coming toward it. Also, note this clever bird (positive pole) looks at events occurring in the inferior surface of the heart in leads II and III. The following strips show what normal events are recorded in leads I, II, and III. Note that the R wave is prominent in these three leads. These form a triangle with the heart at the center (Einthoven's triangle). These leads are also in the frontal plane or the up-and-down, superior-to-inferior look at the heart.

I

II

III

Redrawn from Guyton, Hall: *Textbook of medical physiology,* ed 7, Philadelphia, 1986, Saunders, p. 133.

Do You UNDERSTAND?

DIRECTIONS: **On the following figure, draw leads I, II, and III of a 12-lead ECG and use a positive (+) or negative (−) sign to indicate the appropriate poles.**

Redrawn from Guyton, Hall: Textbook of medical physiology, ed 7, Philadelphia, 1986, Saunders, p. 133.

Answer:

What You NEED TO KNOW

Augmented Leads

The next three leads are also on the frontal surface of the heart. They are called augmented leads and labeled with a small *a*, because the stimulus has to be increased in power to record information from these leads. Augmented leads are also called *unipolar*, because they measure the action of one lead and a body limb.

The last letter in the lead in this system tells you where the positive electrode is placed:

- aV_R records activity from the heart (−) to the right shoulder (+)
- aV_L records activity from the heart (−) to the left shoulder (+)
- aV_F records activity from the heart (−) to the left foot (+)

Redrawn from Copstead, Banasik: Pathophysiology, ed 2, Philadelphia, 2000, Saunders, p. 421.

The following strips show the normal electrical activity recorded in these leads. Again, the smiling lovebird will see events at the bottom of the heart or inferior surface in aV_F, because the positive electrode is looking up from the foot.

| aVR | aVL | aVF |

Redrawn from Copstead, Banasik: Pathophysiology, ed 2, Philadelphia, 2000, Saunders, p. 421.

Do You UNDERSTAND?

DIRECTIONS: **Fill in the blanks for the positive poles of the augmented leads.**

1. aV_R _____

2. aV_L _____

3. aV_F _____

What You NEED TO KNOW

Precordial Leads

The last six leads of a 12-lead ECG look at events in the horizontal plane or surface from the front of the heart toward the patient's back. These are called the precordial or chest leads; they are unipolar leads.

The positive electrode is always in front of the heart, and the negative electrode is the left shoulder. These leads are labeled V_1 through V_6 and are placed across the chest from the right of the sternum to the left axilla.

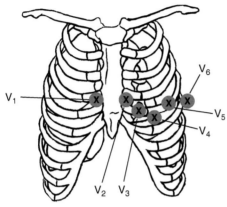

Redrawn from Copstead, Banasik: Pathophysiology, ed 2, Philadelphia, 2000, Saunders, p. 421.

The leads should become progressively more positive as they advance from V_1 through V_6. The first chest lead is V_1, and it is located on the fourth intercostal space (ICS) to the right of the sternum. The second chest lead, V_2, is located next to V1 but to the left of the sternum. Next, we skip V_3 and locate V_4. V_4 is found at the fifth ICS at the midclavicular line or at the point of maximal impulse (PMI). V_3 is found easily now, because it is half way between V_2 and V_4 leads.

V_1 through V_4 are placed so that they look at events occurring in the anterior portion of the left ventricle. V_6 is located next and is found in the left midaxillary line (sixth ICS). V_5 is found half way between V_4 and V_6. Both V_5 and V_6 look at the lateral surface of the left ventricle.

Placement of the precordial leads in the exact location is essential. If they are not correctly placed, important changes in heart activity may be missed.

Do You UNDERSTAND?

DIRECTIONS: **Match the V lead in column A to the definition of its location in column B.**

Column A	Column B
1. _____ V_1	a. Midaxillary line, fifth ICS
2. _____ V_2	b. Fifth ICS, midclavicular line (MCL)
3. _____ V_3	c. Half-way between V_2 and V_4
4. _____ V_4	d. Fourth ICS, right of the sternum
5. _____ V_5	e. Fourth ICS, left of the sternum
6. _____ V_6	f. Half-way between V_4 and V_6

What IS Acute Coronary Syndrome?

Acute coronary syndrome results from ischemia where there is a dangerous imbalance between myocardial oxygen supply and demand, along with the potential for thrombus formation.

What You NEED TO KNOW

Patients may experience chest pain due to myocardial ischemia without developing a myocardial infarction (death of myocardial tissue). In these patients, it is essential to rule out acute MI **first** and then stratify the risk for ischemic heart disease. Protocol-driven management based on evidence-based outcomes is the key to treating patients with ischemic heart disease. Non-modifiable risk factors for coronary artery disease include age, gender, race, and family history of CAD. Modifiable risk factors include smoking, hypertension, sedentary lifestyle, diabetes, obesity, increased alcohol consumption, and stress.

Answers: 1. d; 2. e; 3. c; 4. b; 5. f; 6. a.

What You DO

- Patient presents with chest pain (jaw, arm, epigastric, back, or shoulder pain; unexplained dyspnea, palpitation, or syncope).
- Chest pain triage: Perform history and physical examination—evaluate risk factors, hemodynamic status, and perfusion; perform lung auscultation; evaluate for alternative diagnoses.
- Prompt 12-lead ECG.
- Stratify patient by ECG changes and risk:

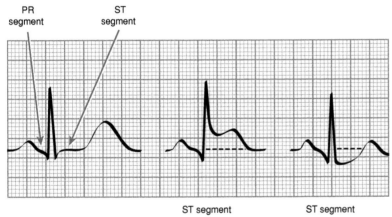

Schumacher, Chernecky: *Real world nursing survival guide:* critical care and emergency nursing, St Louis, 2005, Saunders, pg. 133.

- ST segment elevation meeting fibrinolytic criteria
- ST segment depression 0.05 mm or transient ST segment elevation NOT meeting fibrinolytic criteria (ECG evidence of unstable angina)
- ECG is nondiagnostic or normal
- For ST segment elevation or ST segment depression:

Initial management

- IV access
- Oxygen and pulse oximetry
- Continuous ECG monitoring
- Lab tests—enzymes (troponin I/ CPK MB)

Pharmacologic intervention

- Aspirin 160 to 325 mg PO

- Nitroglycerin sublingual/IV for chest pain
- ß-blockers if not contraindicated
- Morphine sulfate for immediate relief of pain
- Other interventions are based on the length of ischemic symptoms, whether patient meets fibrinolytic criteria, and if cardiac catheterization lab and angioplasty interventions are available.
- For patients who have a nondiagnostic or normal ECG:
  - Initiate ongoing risk-oriented evaluation
  - Assessment and stabilization includes IV access, oxygen and pulse oximetry, continuous ECG monitoring, and repeat biomarker tests
  - Based on risk factors, patient is given a score (Thrombolysis in Myocardial Infarction [TIMI] Trial Risk Score)
  - Interventions are based on risk score
- For further information, see *Saunders Nursing Survival Guide: Critical Care and Emergency Nursing*, Chapter 4, The Cardiovascular System.

Do You UNDERSTAND?

DIRECTIONS: **Fill in the blanks.**

1. Myocardial ischemia is caused by an imbalance of myocardial oxygen _____ and _____.
2. Nonmodifiable risk factors for coronary artery disease include _____, _____, _____, and _____.
3. Modifiable risk factors for CAD include _____, _____, _____, _____, _____, _____, and _____.

What IS a Transmural Infarction?

Now that you can label the leads of a 12-lead ECG, we discuss what you should look for in these areas. In a *transmural infarction*, there are three zones to examine. These areas are sometimes called the current of injury of an infarction. The areas of ischemia, injury, and infarction involve T wave, ST segment, and Q wave changes of the cardiac cycle.

What You NEED TO KNOW

The three zones of injury may not occur immediately. Instead, they may evolve over time. The first zone is the outermost area. This is the area of ischemia and is usually the first to change.

TAKE HOME POINTS

The first zone is an area of reversible ischemia, but if the damage continues, the next zone occurs.

T-wave inversion

Redrawn from Bucher, Melander: *Critical care nursing*, Philadelphia, 1999, Saunders, p. 189.

The T waves usually invert or flip over because of a lack of oxygen and potassium leaking from the damaged heart muscle cells. Remember, normal T waves are upright, larger than P waves, and slightly asymmetric.

Redrawn from Bucher, Melander: *Critical care nursing*, Philadelphia, 1999, Saunders, p. 189.

- The second change to occur is elevation of the ST segment. ST segments are usually isoelectric and need to be greater than 1 mm high to be considered elevated.
- Elevated ST segments indicate prolonged, severe injury to the myocardial cells.
- The ST segments may be elevated so high that the T wave may not be seen until several days later.
- Elevated ST segments indicate acute injury. This is the point at which intervention must take place. They are the first to recede to normal within several days postinfarction.
- If there are Q waves without ST segment elevations, the MI is not acute.

- If some action is not taken by this second change, an infarction can occur.
- Do not wait for Q waves to appear. They suggest that irreversible damage has occurred.
- MIs are diagnosed in conjunction with signs and symptoms, cardiac enzymes, cardiac echocardiography, and cardiac catheterization. The ECG should NEVER be used as the sole basis of diagnosis.

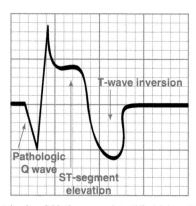

Redrawn from Bucher, Melander: *Critical care nursing*, Philadelphia, 1999, Saunders, p. 189.

- The last change to occur is the Q wave. Taken together, flipped T waves, ST segment elevation, and Q waves are reliable signs (along with cardiac enzymes) that irreversible myocardial necrosis or death has occurred.
- The Q wave must be greater than 0.04 seconds in width and greater than 25% of the height of the R wave to be a pathologic change.
- Treat while there is still some myocardium viable during ST segment elevation!
- Using the ECG alone to diagnose coronary ischemia, injury, or infarction can be complicated due to the amount of myocardial tissue involved in the process. Additionally, the ECGs of patients that have slowed conduction through the left ventricle (left bundle branch block) may be confusing due to the difficulty of detecting ST segment elevation in the presence of left bundle branch block. Therefore serial ECGs, along with serial cardiac enzymes and the clinical presentation of the patient, are used to confirm the diagnosis.

Cardiac enzymes are intracellular enzymes that are released into the blood stream when cell membranes rupture during myocardial infarction. The two enzymes specific for cardiac cellular damage are the CK-MB and troponin I.

There are other enzymes (CPK, LDH, and SGOT) that can be released but are not found exclusively in myocardial tissue and therefore are not specific to myocardial damage.

Cardiac Enzyme Laboratory Findings

Enzyme	Earliest Rise (in hr)	Peak (in hr)	Return to Baseline
CK	2-6	18-36	3-6 days
CK-MB	4-8	15-24	3-4 days
Myoglobin	0.5-1.0	6-9	12 hours
Troponin 1	1-6	7-24	10-14 days

CK, Creatine kinase; *MB*, cardiac muscle marker.
From Schumacher L, Chernecky C: *Real world nursing survival guide: critical care and emergency nursing*, St Louis, 2005, Saunders.

TAKE HOME POINTS

Troponin I is a rapid test that confirms the diagnosis of acute MI, if the serum level is elevated.

Non–Q Wave MI

Occasionally, a patient may show symptoms of an MI with elevated enzymes but a depressed ST segment and no Q waves. This patient may have infarcted the inner part of the muscle wall, the subendocardial surface. Another category of non-Q wave myocardial infarctions include

ST elevation with no Q waves where the patient has incurred damage to the outer surface (subepicardial area) of the heart.

Women wait longer to seek medical attention for symptoms of infarction. Women also have more complications and death with hospitalization, because they are usually older and sicker. Many have other underlying conditions like diabetes and heart failure. Women with high serum uric acid levels after an MI have a poorer prognosis.

Diabetes and hypertension, two leading risk factors for MI, occur more frequently in blacks. Obesity is more common in black women and is a risk factor for coronary atherosclerosis.

What You DO

If you suspect the patient is having an MI, you should remember to do the following:
- Follow the ABCs of airway, breathing, and circulation.
- If the ABCs are present, reassure the patient and ensure that he or she maintains bedrest *(decreases oxygen demand)*.
- Administer oxygen *(increases oxygen supply to the heart)* to keep the SaO_2 greater than 93%.
- *Assess for drug allergies,* and administer sublingual nitroglycerin *based on institutional protocol.*
  The following is based on institutional protocols and physicians' orders:
- Give morphine sulfate at 2 mg intravenously (IV) if three successive sublingual nitroglycerine doses do not abate the patient's chest pain or symptoms.
- Administer aspirin and ß-blockers to the patient. Aspirin has been shown to be effective in decreasing clot formation in patients experiencing MI. α-blockers help reduce the heart rate and decrease oxygen demand on the heart. Bradycardia and hypotension must be ruled out before administering ß-blockers.
- Administer (via IV) nitroglycerin and heparin. Heparin prevents further clot formation and nitroglycerin helps dilate coronary arteries and decrease the workload of the heart by vasodilatation.
- Institute thrombolytic therapy to lyse the clot obstructing the coronary artery if no contraindications. Tissue plasminogen activator (TPA) or its newest version, tenecteplase (TNK) (an enzyme derivative of TPA), may be used, especially if there will be a delay in more definitive therapy.

You must closely observe the patients who show symptoms of an MI with elevated enzymes and ST and T wave changes but no Q waves, because almost 50% of them have infarct damage that extends into the transmural wall.

Ongoing assessments for the signs and symptoms of heart failure, dys-rhythmias, and shock are important.

The health care provider should anticipate further diagnostic studies to be prescribed. Stat cardiac markers or enzymes, electrolytes, and ECG should be requested, and the patient may be prepared for emergency cardiac catheterization, angioplasty, or open-heart surgery for coronary artery bypass grafting (CABG).

TAKE HOME POINTS

In a transmural infarction, the following characteristics are seen:

- **Rate and rhythm:** Can be anything. Rhythm may degrade to ventricular tachycardia (V_T) and ventricular fibrillation (V_F) if untreated.
- **PR interval:** Intervals are normal.
- **QRS complex:** Q waves present in leads looking at the infarction. Qs are greater than 0.04 seconds wide and one fourth the height of the R wave.
- **ST segment:** Segments are elevated greater than 1 mm.
- **QT interval:** Intervals are normal.
- **T wave:** Waves are usually inverted in leads looking at infarcted area.
- **Other:** Because of ventricular irritability, premature ventricular contractions (PVCs) may be present.

Do You UNDERSTAND?

DIRECTIONS: **Fill in the blanks.**

1. The areas of ischemia, injury, and infarction respectively involve _____, _____, and Q-wave changes of the cardiac cycle.
2. The first zone or _____ area is usually the first to change and the area of ischemia; _____ waves invert or flip over because of lack of _____ and _____. Three zones of injury may not occur immediately but evolve over time.
3. If there are Q waves and flipped T waves without ST segment elevations, the MI is not acute but has occurred _____.
4. MIs are diagnosed in conjunction with signs and symptoms, cardiac _____, cardiac echocardiography, and cardiac _____.
5. If the health care provider suspects the patient is having an MI, he or she should first check _____, _____, and _____.

What ARE the Types of Infarction?

Now that you are familiar with all 12 leads and the current treatment of injury for an MI, it is time to discuss the infarction locations and where they can be found. Types of infarction include anterior, inferior, lateral, and posterior, which all refer to the *left ventricle,* because the primary concern is the booster pump to the body.

What You NEED TO KNOW

The size of an MI is determined by how proximal the occlusion is *and the extent of collateral blood flow to the ischemia area.* An anterior infarction is usually the most lethal for the patient, mainly because there is more muscle to lose. In an anterior infarction, the blood supply via the left anterior descending artery has been stopped before reaching the anterior wall of the ventricle. If the left main coronary artery becomes occluded, there is little chance that the patient will survive.

The leads that look at the left ventricle's anterior surface are V_1 through V_4. If this wall of the ventricle has infarcted, you will see Q waves, ST segment elevation, and flipped T waves in the first four V leads.

An inferior MI involves the bottom or diaphragmatic surface of the left ventricle. ECGs suggesting that the patient has suffered an MI would have three changes in leads II, III, and aV_F. Inferior wall MIs are caused by blockages in the right coronary artery (RCA). Often patients suffering from inferior MIs have heart blocks, because the RCA supplies the sinoatrial (SA) and atrioventricular (AV) nodes in a large percentage of the population.

A lateral wall infarction of the left ventricle is confirmed by looking in lead I, aV_L, V_5, and V_6. The circumflex artery supplies the lateral wall of the ventricle.

Isolated posterior wall MIs are very rare. Additional electrodes can be added to the 12 leads on the patient's back at V_7 (posterior axillary line), V_8 (midscapular line), and V_9 (3 cm from the spinal column). In addition, reciprocal (opposite) changes in the chest leads can be examined. In V_1 and V_2, the R wave is usually at its lowest voltage. Reciprocal changes in these leads suggest a posterior wall MI, indicated by tall R waves in V_1 and V_2 (opposite of deep Qs), ST segment depression, and high, peaked T waves.

Studies show that a woman's susceptibility to anterior infarction leading to mortality rises after menopause.

Anterior MI

Redrawn from Huszar: *Pocket guide to basic dysrhythmias,* ed 2, St Louis, 1995, Mosby, p. 80. Arrows indicate ST elevation.

Inferior MI

Redrawn from Bucher, Melander: *Critical care nursing*, Philadelphia, 1999, Saunders, p. 191.

What You DO

When checking for the 12-lead ECG for evidence of an infarction, you should do the following:

- Look in the V leads first (these are the most dangerous).
- Look in the inferior leads next (II, III, aV_F).
- Look in the lateral leads next (I, aV_L, V_5, V_6).
- Examine V_1 and V_2 for tall R waves, ST segment depression, and tall T waves.

To summarize which leads look at what surfaces, examine the following table:

Electrocardiographic Changes Localizing a Myocardial Infarction

Location of MI	Indicative Changes*	Reciprocal Changes†	Affected Coronary Artery
Lateral	I, aV$_L$, V$_5$, V$_6$	V$_1$-V$_3$	Left coronary artery—circumflex branch
Inferior	II, III, aV$_F$	I, aV$_L$	Right coronary artery—posterior descending branch
Septum	V$_1$, V$_2$	None	Left coronary artery—left anterior descending artery, septal branch
Anterior	V$_3$, V$_4$	II, III, aV$_F$	Left coronary artery—left anterior descending artery, diagonal branch
Posterior	Not visualized	V$_1$, V$_2$, V$_3$, V$_4$	Right coronary artery or left circumflex artery
Right ventricle	V$_1$R-V$_6$R		Right coronary artery—proximal branches

*Leads facing affected areas.
†Leads opposite affected areas.
From Aehlert B: *ECGs made easy*, ed 2, St Louis, 2002, Mosby.

Do You UNDERSTAND?

DIRECTIONS: **What type of MI does the strip on the following page represent?**

1. _____

Redrawn from Huszar: *Pocket guide to basic dysrhthmias,* ed 2, St Louis, 1995, Mosby, p. 84.

References

Aehlert B: *ECGs made easy,* ed 2, St Louis, 2002, Mosby.

American Heart Association: *Advanced cardiac life support provider manual,* Dallas, 1997, American Heart Association.

Bucher L: Acute myocardial infarction. In Bucher L, Melander S: *Critical care nursing,* Philadelphia, 1999, Saunders.

Ehrat K: *The art of EKG interpretation,* ed 4, Dubuque, IA, 1997, Kendall-Hunt.

Halm M, Penque S: Heart disease in women, *Am J Nurs* 99(4):26, 1999.

Miracle V, Sims J: Making sense of the 12-lead ECG, *Nursing* 29(7):34, 1999.

O'Donnell M, Dirks J: Cardiovascular disorders. In Urden L, Stacy K: *Priorities in critical care nursing,* ed 3, St Louis, 2000, Mosby.

Perrin KQ: Interventions for critically ill patients with coronary artery disease. In Ignatavicius DD, Workman M, Mishler M: *Medical-surgical nursing across the health care continuum,* vol 1, ed 3, Philadelphia, 1999, Saunders.

NCLEX® Review

1. You are instructing a UAP to perform a 12-lead ECG. You know he or she is learning correct lead placement when he or she says:
   1 "All of the limb leads go across the chest."
   2 "V_6 is positioned under the left armpit, just above the last two ribs."
   3 "Accuracy isn't really important when placing the precordial leads."
   4 "V_1 is at the left of the sternum in the fourth intercostal space."

2. A patient is said to have had a transmural infarction when he has a:
   1 QRS between 0.10 and 0.12
   2 Prolonged PR interval
   3 High-peaked T wave
   4 Q wave one fourth the depth of the R wave

3. The precordial leads are:
   1 I, II, and III
   2 aV_R, aV_L, aV_F
   3 II, III, and aV_F
   4 V_1 through V_6

4. The earliest sign on the ECG that an infarction is occurring is:
   1 A wide Q wave
   2 ST segment depression
   3 T-wave elevation
   4 T-wave depression

NCLEX® Review Answers

1. 2 V_6 is in the fifth intercostal space at the midaxillary line. Not all 12 leads go across the chest. Lead placement is of the utmost importance because if placed incorrectly they can cause error in readings by the health care provider. V_2, not V_1, is at the left of the sternum in the fourth intercostal space.

2. 4 A transmural infarction causes the loss of the R wave and a deep Q wave that is more than one fourth the height of the patient's R wave. A QRS between .10 and .12 is not long enough for a transmural Q wave. A prolonged PR interval is characteristic of a heart block, not an infarction. T-wave inversion is a characteristic of an infarction.

3. 4 The V leads are also called precordial leads and go across the left chest, from the right of the heart to the left. I, II, and III are limb leads. aV_R, aV_L, and aV_F are augmented leads. II, III, and aV_F look at the inferior surface of the left ventricle.

4. 4 T waves flip over, indicating ischemia of myocardial cells. The Q wave is generally the last sign to appear because necrosis takes several hours to evolve. ST depression will occur in the leads opposite of the infarction. T-wave depression is a sign of ischemia, which is the first zone of an infarction.

Notes

Pericarditis and Cardiac Tamponade

Chapter

20

What You WILL LEARN

After reading this chapter, you will know how to do the following:
- ✔ Define pericarditis.
- ✔ Describe cardiac tamponade.
- ✔ List two possible causes of cardiac tamponade.

What IS Pericarditis?

Pericarditis is an inflammation of the heart sac (**pericardium**). The pericardium is a double-layered membrane lining the heart. The outer layer is called the *pericardium,* and the inner layer is called the *epicardium.* The potential space between the two layers contains 30 to 50 mL of serous, lubricating fluid.

Viral infections (e.g., coxsackievirus, varicella, influenza, HIV) and bacterial infections (e.g., tuberculosis [TB]) are the most common causes of this inflammation. Uremia, renal failure, rheumatic fever, posttraumatic pericarditis, and connective tissue diseases (systemic lupus erythematosus, scleroderma, and rheumatoid arthritis) may also cause pericarditis.

Pericarditis can also be caused by medications such as procainamide and hydralazine; radiation treatment for Hodgkin's disease, breast cancer, leukemia, or lymphoma; tumor metastasis to the heart from lung cancer, breast cancer, leukemia, or lymphoma; and by cardiac trauma related to surgery, blunt trauma, or penetrating trauma (see Chapter 23).

305

Sometimes pericarditis is the result of a myocardial infarction (MI) across all muscle layers of the heart (**transmural infarction**). The dead and ischemic tissues in an MI stimulate the body's immune response to send white cells and fibrin deposits to the area producing fluid exudates, which tend to irritate and inflame the pericardium. Any fluid accumulation in the pericardial cavity is called **pericardial effusion**. This fluid exudate can accumulate in large enough amounts to lead to compression of the heart, causing a decrease in cardiac output. This emergent condition is called *cardiac tamponade.*

What IS Cardiac Tamponade?

Cardiac tamponade is the progressive accumulation of fluid in the pericardial sac causing increased intracardiac pressures and compression of the atria and ventricles. The fluid can be blood, transudative or, more often, an exudate. As intrapericardial pressure rises during cardiac tamponade (more fluid builds up in the sac), right ventricular filling decreases, and less blood is delivered to the lungs. Ultimately this decreased blood flow leads to less blood going to the left ventricle, which decreases stroke volume. As a result, the pericardial heart sac stretches to accommodate the increased fluid. This causes increased heart rate, peripheral constriction, and sodium and water retention. If the fluid accumulates too rapidly or in too large a quantity, the pericardial fluid pressure will equal diastolic pressures, leading to a severe decrease in stroke volume and circulatory collapse. The end result is hypoperfusion of all organs.

What You NEED TO KNOW

The classic presentation of pericarditis is chest pain, which worsens on inspiration (**pleuritic pain**) or when lying down. This pain is described as sharp with abrupt onset. The pain lessens when the patient sits up and leans forward.

When listening to the heart, a scratchy sound is also present. This is called a friction rub and is caused by the roughened surfaces of the heart's layers rubbing over one another. The heart sounds may become distant if enough fluid is present.

Classic signs of cardiac tamponade include elevated central venous pressure (CVP) with neck vein distension, distant heart sounds, and arterial hypotension; these are known as Beck's triad. Other findings include dyspnea, tachycardia, and electrical alternans on the electrocardiogram (ECG) (the height of the QRS complex changes with each successive beat, or it is alternately increased and then decreased). Pulsus paradoxus (PP) may also be present. PP is the decrease in systolic blood pressure by greater than 10 mm Hg during inspiration. It can be identified as the pulse becomes palpably weaker during inspiration and stronger during expiration.

A 12-lead ECG may show the following during pericarditis and cardiac tamponade:

Redrawn from Bucher, Melander: *Critical care nursing*, Philadelphia, 1999, Saunders, p. 295.

- Sinus rhythm or sinus tachycardia.
- PR interval of the ECG may be depressed but of normal duration.
- Voltage of the QRS complex may be low.
- QRS complexes may alternate voltage with each beat in a large-small pattern. In other words, one complex is taller, the next is smaller, the next is taller, and so on. This is known as electrical alternans and may indicate that large amounts of fluid are compressing the heart's blood inflow (cardiac tamponade).

- ST segment is elevated as with an MI; however, it is elevated throughout all of the leads of the ECG. Unlike an MI, pericarditis involves the whole heart, not different locations of the heart.
- Q waves do not occur.
- ST segment has a saggy or concave appearance.
- QT interval time is not affected by pericarditis; however, the T wave is upright initially.
- In the recovery phase, the T wave inverts.

The following table shows the differences between ECG changes in an MI versus pericarditis.

ECG Changes

	Myocardial Infarction	Pericarditis
PR interval	Can prolong block	Unchanged into heart
QRS complex	Q waves	No Q waves
ST segment	Elevated only in affected leads	Elevated with concave ST segment in all leads
QT interval	Longer in inferior MI	Unchanged
T wave	Inverted in leads looking at the infarction	Upright in all leads, then inverted in all

MI, Myocardial infarction.

Differences in laboratory values in MI versus pericarditis include (1) elevated erythrocyte sedimentation rate (ESR) caused by inflammation process in pericarditis, and (2) pericardial fluid analysis that reveals lower fibrinogen and hematocrit values than the peripheral blood values in pericarditis.

What You DO

When treating patients with pericarditis, you should do the following:
- Position the patient in semi-Fowler's position.
- Auscultate the left lower sternal border where the pericardium lies and where you can best hear a pericardial friction rub (high-pitched scratchy sound heard at the end of inspiration).
- Anticipate possible performance of an echocardiogram (ECHO) to confirm the diagnosis of pericarditis. An ECHO is a noninvasive test

performed at the bedside that uses Doppler technology to check the heart and underlying structures.

- Position the patient who has precordial pain in a comfortable position, which is usually sitting upright or leaning forward over the bedside table.
- Assess for increased CVP via a central or pulmonary artery catheter line.
- Assess for pulsus paradoxus, dyspnea, and low urine output.
- Administer oxygen if the SaO_2 is less than 93%.
- Administer prescribed drugs. Analgesics, such as salicylates and codeine and nonsteroidal antiinflammatory drugs (NSAIDs) are commonly used to decrease pain and inflammation. Prednisone can be prescribed for severe acute pericarditis but not if the cause is TB, because prednisone exacerbates TB.
- Target treatment toward the underlying cause of the pericarditis, such as antibiotics for bacterial infections.
- Remember that most patients recover within a few weeks.

If you must assist with a pericardiocentesis, you should have an ECG machine on standby. The needle used to remove the fluid from the pericardial sac is attached to the ECG machine with a special clamp. The needle then becomes the electrode. The health care provider pulls the needle back when the ECG shows ST segment elevation, indicating the needle is in the myocardium. Aspiration is then performed.

If the pericardiocentesis is successful, the results to the patient are generally immediate and dramatic. The patient's heart sounds become clearer, the blood pressure (BP) rises, and the neck veins become flat. Sometimes a small chest catheter or chest tube is inserted and left in place, especially if it is thought that fluid will build up again. Sometimes a sclerosing agent (bleomycin, cisplatin, tetracycline) is instilled into the pericardial space to produce an inflammatory response that closes up the space.

In addition, surgery (a pericardial window) can be performed to remove a small piece (a few centimeters) of pericardium to allow the fluid to drain out.

Cardiac tamponade is a medical emergency. Immediately notify the health care provider and prepare for a pericardiocentesis (insertion of a needle under the xyphoid process into the pericardial sac to withdraw the fluid) if the patient develops muffled heart sounds, distended neck veins, and a rapidly decreasing blood pressure (Beck's triad) and /or pulsus paradoxus.

Do You UNDERSTAND?

DIRECTIONS: **List the causes of pericarditis.**

1. Viral causes

   _____
   _____
   _____
   _____

2. Other causes

   _____
   _____
   _____
   _____
   _____
   _____
   _____
   _____
   _____
   _____
   _____
   _____

DIRECTIONS: **Place a check mark in front of the signs and symptoms of pericarditis.**

3. a. _____ Dull, achy pain
   b. _____ Sharp, stabbing pain
   c. _____ Pain worsening on expiration
   d. _____ Pain eases with leaning forward
   e. _____ Distant muffled heart sounds
   f. _____ Cardiac friction rub

DIRECTIONS: **Fill in the blanks.**

4. The classic sign of cardiac tamponade when the patient's pulse becomes weaker during inspiration is called _____

   _____.

5. The noninvasive test that will tell if the patient has pericarditis is

   _____.

6. The position of comfort to decrease pain from pericarditis is

   _____.

7. Two drugs given to decrease inflammation from pericarditis are
   _____ and _____.

8. If the SaO$_2$ is less than 93%, _____ is
   administered.

9. Three signs and symptoms (Beck's triad) that signal a pericarditis
   may be changing into cardiac tamponade are _____,
   _____, and _____.

10. Auscultation of the pericardium is best at what anatomic location?
    _____

11. Prednisone should not be administered to patient's with
    pericarditis who have what other disease?

    _____

References

Anderson K, editor: *Mosby's medical, nursing and allied health dictionary,* ed 5,
   St Louis, 1998, Mosby.

Barach P: Pulsus paradoxus. In *Hospital physician,* Wayne, PA, 2000, Turner White
   Communications.

Brashers VL: Alterations in cardiovascular functions. In McCance KL, Huether SE,
   editors: *Pathophysiology: the biologic basis for disease in adults and children,* ed 4,
   St Louis, 2002, Mosby.

Chernecky C, Berger B: *Laboratory tests and diagnostic procedures,* ed 3, Philadelphia,
   2001, Saunders.

Copstead LEC, Banasik JC: *Pathophysiology: biological and behavioral perspectives,* ed
   2, Philadelphia, 2000, Saunders.

Davenport J, Morton PG: Identifying nonischemic causes of life-threatening
   arrhythmias, *Am J Nurs* 97(11):50, 1997.

Ehrat K: *The art of EKG interpretation: a self-instructional text,* ed 4, Dubuque, IA,
   1997, Kendal Hunt.

Khasnis A, Lokhandwala Y: Clinical signs in medicine: pulsus paradoxus, *J Postgrad
   Med* 48:46-49, 2002.

Lamborn ML, Moseley MJ: Cardiac alterations. In Hartshorn JC, Sole ML,
   Lamborn ML, editors: *Introduction to critical care nursing,* ed 3, Philadelphia,
   2001, Saunders.

McCoy C, Livingston N: Cardiovascular laboratory and diagnostic tests. In Bucher
   L, Melander S: *Critical care nursing,* Philadelphia, 1999, Saunders.

Skidmore L: *Mosby's drug guide for nurses,* St Louis, 2001, Mosby.

Thelan LA et al: *Critical care nursing: diagnosis and management,* ed 3, St Louis,
   1998, Mosby.

Answers: 7, NSAIDs, salicylates; 8, oxygen; 9, muffled heart sounds, rapidly decreasing blood pressure, distended neck veins; 10, left lower sternal border; 11, tuberculosis (TB).

NCLEX® Review

1. Which of the following is not a viral cause of peri-carditis?
   1 Liver cancer
   2 Varicella
   3 Influenza
   4 Coxsackie

2. In cardiac tamponade, cardiac output is:
   1 Increased
   2 Decreased
   3 Within normal limits
   4 Only affected if accompanied by hypotension

3. Pleuritic chest pain as a symptom of pericarditis worsens:
   1 During inspiration
   2 During expiration
   3 While sitting up
   4 While leaning forward

4. Your nursing assessment for a patient with probable cardiac tamponade reveals that pulses become weaker during inspiration. This sign is called:
   1 Electrical alternans
   2 Tachycardia
   3 Precordial friction rib
   4 Pulsus paradoxus

5. Electrical alternans in an ECG is assessed in what part of the ECG cycle?
   1 T wave
   2 P wave
   3 PR interval
   4 QRS complex

6. Pericarditis is an inflammatory process that increases what laboratory value?
   1 Hematocrit (HCT)
   2 Total red blood cell (RBC) count
   3 Erythrocyte sedimentation rate (ESR)
   4 Prothrombin time (PT)

7. A pericardial friction rub is best auscultated:
   1 Over the second intercostal space, right midclavicular line (MCL)
   2 Two finger breaths to the right of the xyphoid process at the fourth intercostal space
   3 Over the mid–xyphoid process
   4 Over the left lower sternal border

8. Withdrawal of fluid from the pericardial sac is known as a(n):
   1 Echocardiogram
   2 Pericardiocentesis
   3 Xyphoid endoscopy
   4 Thoracentesis

9. Which of the following is an indication of a successful pericardiocentesis?
   1 Hypotension
   2 Cardiac standstill
   3 Clearer heart sounds to auscultation
   4 Increased temperature

NCLEX® Review Answers

1. 1 Liver cancer is not a virus. Varicella, influenza, and *Coxsackie* are all viruses that can precipitate pericarditis.

2. 2 Cardiac tamponade decreases cardiac output. Fluid build-up does compress the heart. Cardiac output is not only affected if accompanied by hypotension; it is affected by multiple factors, such as decreased stroke volume and increased heart rate.

3. 1 Pleuritic pain worsens on inspiration because this increases pressure within the thoracic cavity and on the heart itself. Pleuritic pain lessens when the patient is sitting or leaning forward.

4. 4 When pulses become weaker during inspiration in a patient with cardiac tamponade, it is known as pulsus paradoxus. Electrical alternans is a phenomenon seen on the ECG strip. Tachycardia would be a fast heart rate and pulse, not a weak one. Precordial friction rub is a high-pitched sound heard on auscultation at the end of inspiration.

5. 4 Electrical alternans can be assessed from the QRS complex on the ECG because the QRS alternates voltage. The T wave, P wave, and PR interval do not help assess electrical alternans.

6. 3 Pericarditis should increase the laboratory values for ESR because this increases with inflammation. HCT is associated with the percentage of red blood cells in volume. Total RBC count is associated with numbers of red blood cells, whereas PT is associated with clotting.

7. 4 The pericardium lies at the left lower sternal border, and therefore a pericardial friction rub is best auscultated here.

8. 2 Pericardiocentesis. An echocardiogram is a noninvasive ultrasound procedure of the heart. Thoracentesis is the removal of fluid from the lungs, not the pericardial sac. There is no such procedure as a xyphoid endoscopy.

9. 3 Clearer heart sounds on auscultation, increased blood pressure, and distended neck veins are indications of a successful pericardiocentesis. Hypotension could be a sign of cardiac perforation. If cardiac standstill occurs, CPR should be initiated immediately. Increased temperature would be a sign of infection.

Notes

Chapter 21

Drug Effects, Toxicities, and Electrolytes

What You WILL LEARN

After reading this chapter, you will know how to do the following:

✔ Describe the effect of Digoxin (Lanoxin) on the heart.
✔ Define a Class IA antidysrhythmic.
✔ Describe when a ß-blocker would be prescribed.
✔ Define calcium channel blocker.
✔ Differentiate hypokalemia from hyperkalemia.
✔ Describe the symptoms and signs of hypocalcemia.
✔ Describe one electrocardiogram change seen in hypercalcemia.
✔ Define hypomagnesemia.
✔ Differentiate hypermagnesemia from hypomagnesemia.

Drugs can have a striking effect on the waveforms of an electrocardiogram (ECG). Some medications (digoxin, procainamide, quinidine) can alter normal patterns. In addition, changes on the ECG can help determine whether patients are developing toxicity from their medications. Serum electrolyte level changes can also show up on the ECG; occasionally, the health care provider can observe changes before serum level reports are back. Therefore it is important for you to know how drugs and electrolytes cause ECG changes.

For further information see *Saunders Nursing Survival Guide: Pharmacology,* Chapter 5, Drugs Affecting the Cardiac System.

What IS Digoxin?

Digoxin (Lanoxin, Lanoxicaps) is a widely used drug that slows the transportation of sodium and potassium across the heart cell membrane. Digoxin is in a class of drugs called the cardiac glycosides; it slows the influx of sodium and allows an influx of calcium that helps the cardiac muscles to contract. This leads to greater contracting strength of the myocardial cells **(positive inotropy)**. Because the heart is a more efficient pump, it causes an increase in cardiac output.

Digoxin also slows the heart rate **(negative chronotropic effect)** and atrioventricular (AV) conduction **(negative dromotropic effect)**. This effect can be beneficial in slowing fast rhythms; however, if the heart rate slows too much, low cardiac output results.

What You NEED TO KNOW

Digoxin is used to increase cardiac contractility; it is often used in heart failure to improve cardiac output. Digoxin can be used to slow down fast cardiac rhythms, such as atrial fibrillation and flutter. It does this by slowing down AV conduction. Digoxin can cause a slurring or scooping of the ST segment. Sometimes the T wave will be lost in this scooping effect.

Redrawn from Lipman, Lipman: *ECG pocket guide,* St Louis, 1987, Mosby, p.120.

 TAKE HOME POINTS

Digoxin can have a depressive effect that causes bradycardia and heart block. Excessive digitalis can result in any type of abnormal heart rhythm, including those with slower heart rates (junctional rhythms, heart blocks) or those with faster atrial rates (atrial tachycardia with block). Other signs of the effect of digoxin on the heart that you can see on the ECG strip include the following:
- **PR interval:** May be prolonged (> 0.20 seconds)
- **ST segment:** May have a scooped effect
- **QT interval:** May be shortened
- **T wave:** May fuse into the ST segment

Digitalis can cause the QT interval to shorten and the PR interval to prolong. Dysrhythmias thought to be caused by digitalis toxicity or excess are diagnosed clinically and not strictly from the ECG. The following conditions can increase the chance of developing higher than normal digoxin levels:

Conditions that Increase Digoxin Toxicity

- Hypokalemia
- Hypercalcemia
- Renal impairment
- Advanced age
- Acute hypoxia
- Hypothyroidism
- Drug use of amphotericin B, quinidine, amiodarone, diltiazem, captopril, furosemide, erythromycin, ibuprofen, nifedipine, and/or verapamil
- Herbal use of cascara sagrada bark, ginseng, pleurisy root, ephedra (ma huang), ephedrine, and/or sarsaparilla

Hypokalemia is a common culprit that causes digitoxicity even if the digoxin level is normal. Therefore you should monitor the patients' potassium level and watch for signs of weakness.

TAKE HOME POINTS

- Digoxin has a very narrow therapeutic margin of 0.5 to 1.5 mg/dL, and it is excreted from the body slowly.
- Serum digoxin levels need to be monitored, especially in older patients.

What You DO

When treating patients who are receiving digitalis, you should perform the following:
- Monitor serum digoxin levels or remind the health care provider to order a digitalis level.
- Withhold the digoxin dose if digitalis toxicity is suspected and report to the health care provider.
- Monitor for signs of toxicity that include abnormal heart rhythms, visual disturbances (green or yellow halos around objects), and gastrointestinal symptoms (nausea, vomiting, diarrhea).
- Monitor for conditions that increase toxicity.
- Administer lidocaine and phenytoin (Dilantin) to counteract abnormal ventricular rhythms caused by digoxin.
- Administer digoxin immune Fab (Digibind) to reverse life-threatening digitoxicity. However, Digibind is expensive. If the patient has normal

kidney function and the dysrhythmias associated with the digitoxicity are not life-threatening, the digitalis can be eliminated without medication.

Do You UNDERSTAND?

DIRECTIONS: **Complete the following exercises.**

1. List two ways that digoxin improves the pumping action of the heart.

   _____

   _____

2. What are the potentially negative effects of digoxin?

   _____

   _____

DIRECTIONS: **Fill in the blanks.**

3. The normal therapeutic range for serum digoxin is _____ to _____ mg/dL.

4. Digoxin has a _____ effect on the ST segment.

5. Electrolyte imbalances that can cause digitalis toxicity include _____ and _____ .

6. _____ , _____ , and _____ cardiac rhythms can be caused by too much digoxin.

7. Do not give digoxin to patients with _____ , _____ , and _____ heart rhythms.

• Toxicity can cause a variety of undesirable disturbances. Premature ventricular contractions (PVCs), heart blocks, and ventricular tachycardia can be digoxin induced.

• Do not give digoxin to patients with heart blocks, sick sinus syndrome, or Wolff-Parkinson-White syndrome with atrial fibrillation or flutter. The treatment of patients with accessory atrioventricular pathways and paroxysmal supraventricular tachycardia (PSVT) is usually direct-current cardioversion.

• Quinidine can double digoxin levels. Consult the prescribing health care provider if both drugs are ordered. The digitalis dose may be cut in half.

What IS a Class IA Antidysrhythmic?

Class IA antidysrhythmics are a group of drugs that include procainamide (Pronestyl-SR, Procan SR), quinidine (Quinoline, Quinaglute) and disopyramide (e.g., Norpace). These drugs slow entrance of sodium into

Answers: **1. increases contractility; slows conduction in fast-heart rhythms. 2.** If a patient on digoxin already has a slow heart rate, low cardiac output can result. **3.** 0.5, 1.5; **4.** scooping; **5.** hypokalemia, hypercalcemia; **6.** PVCs, heart blocks, ventricular tachycardia; **7.** heart block, sick sinus syndrome, Wolff-Parkinson-White syndrome.

the cardiac cell and thus decrease the rate of depolarization. These medications depress ectopic areas in both atria and ventricles.

What You NEED TO KNOW

Class IA antidysrhythmic drugs slow down both atrial and ventricular rates. They do not affect rhythm but will prolong atrioventricular conduction. When patients receive antidysrhythmic drugs, the ECG may show a slight widening of the QRS complex and a lengthening of the QT interval.

Normal

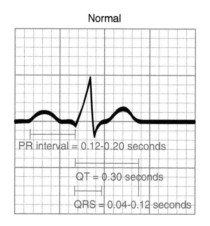

PR interval = 0.12-0.20 seconds

QT = 0.30 seconds

QRS = 0.04-0.12 seconds

Class IA Antidysrhythmics

U wave

PR > normal 0.12 seconds

QT > 0.44 seconds

QRS = 0.12 seconds

In toxicity, heart block can develop, and the QT interval can prolong even further. The rate may become so slow that sometimes another small, positive, upright wave (U wave) occurs after the T wave. A U wave is thought to be caused by repolarization of the Purkinje fibers.

Torsades de pointes is a variant type of ventricular tachycardia (V_T); the wide QRS in this rhythm twists and turns above and below the baseline (see Chapter 13).

⚠ If the QT interval prolongs more than one half the preceding R-to-R time, the patient may develop torsades de pointes.

Redrawn from Bucher, Melander: *Critical care nursing*, Philadelphia, 1999, Saunders, p. 185.

What You DO

- Be prepared to administer magnesium and institute cardiac pacing to override this abnormal stimulus electronically and slow down the heart rate if torsades de pointes occurs.
- Observe the patient's ECG closely for excessive prolongation of the PR interval, QRS complex, and QT and RR intervals.
- Hold the drug, and notify the health care provider, if the QT prolongs more than one half the RR.
- Monitor for signs and symptoms of gastrointestinal effects, such as nausea, vomiting, and diarrhea.

TAKE HOME POINTS

Class IA antidysrhythmics may affect the ECG in the following ways:
- **Rate:** Decreased atrial and ventricular rates
- **Rhythm:** No effect
- **PR interval:** Longer than normal
- **QRS complex:** May widen (usually around 0.12 seconds)
- **QT interval:** Longer than normal (greater than 0.44 seconds)
- **Other:** Development of a U wave

Do You UNDERSTAND?

DIRECTIONS: **Indicate in the spaces provided whether the following statements are *true* or *false*.**

1. _____ Class 1A antidysrhythmics block the renin and angiotension cycle.
2. _____ Class 1A antidysrhythmics do not affect the rhythm, but they will prolong conduction.
3. _____ In toxic doses, Class 1A antidysrhythmics can cause prolongation of the QT interval and heart block.
4. _____ Class 1A antidysrhythmics may cause a U wave to occur.
5. _____ The U wave is thought to be stimulation of the His bundle.

Monitor the patient who is taking Pronestyl for lupus-like syndromes, which may start as rash, fatigue, and swollen achy joints. Also, watch for bleeding.

Answers: **1. false; 2. true; 3. true; 4. true; 5. false.**

DIRECTIONS: **Match the term in column A with the definition in column B.**

Column A	Column B
6. _____ U wave	a. Pronestyl, quinidine, and Norpace
7. _____ Torsades de pointes	b. Trouble if prolongs more than one half the R-R
8. _____ Lupus	c. Longer than 0.20 seconds
9. _____ PR interval	d. Positive deflection between T and P waves
10. _____ Magnesium	e. Rash; fatigue; and swollen, achy joints
11. _____ Cardiac pacing	f. Treatment for torsades de pointes
12. _____ QT interval	g. Greater than 0.44 seconds
	h. Twisting of the QRS around the baseline

What IS a ß-Blocker?

Beta blockers are commonly prescribed drugs that are used to control blood pressure (BP) and to slow down the heart rate in fast rhythms. ß-blockers work by blocking the action of the sympathetic nervous system (SNS); that is, they block the fight-or-flight response of circulating catecholamines. The desired effect is decreased oxygen demand on the heart. These drugs belong to the class II antidysrhythmic drugs. Commonly used drugs in this class are metoprolol (Lopressor), acebutolol (Sectral), esmolol (Brevibloc), and sotalol (Betapace).

Answers: 6, d; 7, h; 8, e; 9, c; 10, f; 11, a; 12, g.

What You NEED TO KNOW

ß-blockers work by slowing down the sinoatrial (SA) node rate. They also slow down conduction. The PR interval may be slightly prolonged, and the QT interval may be shortened.

TAKE HOME POINTS

Generic ß-blockers may be distinguished by other drug classes by name; most of the generic names end in *olol*.

What You DO

When treating patients receiving ß-blockers, you should do the following:
- Monitor the patient's heart rate, BP, and ECG.
- Pay particular attention to the duration of the QRS; hold the drug and notify the health care provider if the QRS expands 25% (when compared with previous width).
- Monitor serum electrolytes and correct any imbalances before starting ß-blockers.
- Remember that symptoms of asthma or bronchospasm can occur in some patients because drugs in this class have pulmonary effects.
- Avoid this medication if the patient is bradycardic, in heart block, or is hypotensive.
- Remember that ß-blockers decrease contractility; however, there are selective ß-blockers that can be used in heart failure.

TAKE HOME POINTS

ß-blockers may affect the ECG in the following ways:
- **Rates:** Slows the heart rate
- **Rhythm:** May cause heart blocks
- **PR interval:** May prolong PR interval
- **QRS complex:** If widening of greater than 25% occurs, the dose should be decreased
- **QT interval:** Shortens the QT interval

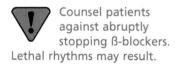

Counsel patients against abruptly stopping ß-blockers. Lethal rhythms may result.

- Observe the patient for signs and symptoms of heart failure, especially when used in combination with other drugs (digoxin) that also slow the heart rate.

Do You UNDERSTAND?

DIRECTIONS: **Indicate in the spaces provided whether the following statements are *true* or *false*.**

1. _____ Before starting therapy with ß-blockers, serum electrolytes should be corrected.
2. _____ You should monitor the patient for signs of heart failure when they are taking ß-blockers.
3. _____ ß-blockers work by slowing down the amount of calcium entering the cardiac cells.
4. _____ ß-blockers shorten the PR and QT intervals.
5. _____ A widening of the QRS complex of more than 25% is an expected outcome of ß-blocker therapy.

What IS a Calcium Channel Blocker?

Calcium channel blockers are drugs given to lower the BP in patients with hypertension. They also slow down the heart rate in fast rhythms (e.g., atrial tachycardia, atrial flutter, atrial fibrillation).

What You NEED TO KNOW

Calcium channel blockers work by slowing down the influx of calcium into the cardiac cell, thus decreasing the contractility of the cell. They are in a class of drugs known as class IV antidysrhythmics. Some of the drugs in this class are verapamil (Calan), nifedipine (Procardia), and diltiazem (Cardizem).

Answers: 1. True, 2. True, 3. False, 4. False, 5. False.

Calcium channel blockers are most commonly used for supraventricular tachycardias (SVTs) because of their ability to slow AV nodal conduction time and prolong AV nodal refractory time.

What You DO

When treating patients who are receiving calcium channel blockers, you should do the following:

- Monitor the patient's heart rate, BP, and ECG when starting calcium channel blockers.
- Advise the patient to rise slowly from a resting position. Calcium channel blockers can cause postural hypotension.
- Consult the health care provider if dizziness or postural hypotension continues. The dose may need to be changed.

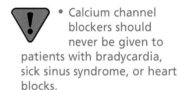

- Calcium channel blockers should never be given to patients with bradycardia, sick sinus syndrome, or heart blocks.
- The patient can have adverse effects to calcium channel blockers that include bradycardia, heart failure, and hypotension.

Do You UNDERSTAND?

DIRECTIONS: Fill in the blanks.

1. Calcium channel blockers work by _____ down the influx of calcium into the cardiac cell, thus _____ the contractility of the cell.

2. The patient can experience adverse effects from calcium channel blockers that include _____, _____, and _____.

TAKE HOME POINTS
Calcium channel blockers can cause the following ECG changes:
- **Rates:** Slowed from previous rate
- **PR interval:** May be prolonged
- **QT interval:** May be prolonged

Electrolyte Effects

Serum and tissue electrolyte imbalances most frequently associated with ECG changes include abnormal potassium, calcium, and magnesium levels (see *Real World Nursing Survival Guide: Fluids & Electrolytes,* Chapters 5, 7, and 8). Normal electrolyte values vary; therefore it is important to check the "normals" for the institution. In general, blood levels of these electrolytes in adults are as follows:

Answers: 1. slowing, decreasing 2. bradycardia, heart failure, hypotension.

- Potassium = 3.5 to 5.2 mEq/L
- Calcium = 8.5 to 11 mg/dL
- Magnesium = 1.5 to 2 mEq/L

TAKE HOME POINTS

The most common cause of hypokalemia is potassium-wasting diuretics.

What IS Hypokalemia?

Hypokalemia is a potassium level of below 3.5 mEq/L. The loss of potassium can lead to PVCs, V_T, and ventricular fibrillation (V_F).

What You NEED TO KNOW

Hypokalemia can be caused by conditions that remove potassium from the body. Although many drugs can do this, the most common culprits are digoxin (Lanoxin); potassium-wasting diuretics, such as furosemide (Lasix), and corticosteroids (Solu-Cortef).

Potassium can also be lost from the urine in patients with elevated blood glucose levels.

Hypokalemia can also be created by conditions that decrease potassium from coming into the body. Dieting, decreased dietary ingestion of potassium, and vomiting can lead to this condition. Serum potassium levels can also be decreased by diarrhea and gastric suctioning.

The diagnosis of hypokalemia is never made on ECG changes alone. It must always be confirmed with a serum potassium level before treatment. A potassium below 3.5 can cause the following ECG changes to the normal waveform:

- ST segment: Depressed
- QT interval: Prolonged
- T wave: Decreased amplitude
- U waves: Present (if a U wave is present, the QT interval is measured to the end of the U wave and is sometimes called the QU interval)

Normal

Hypokalemia

U wave

ST-segment depression

Untreated hypokalemia can lead to PVCs, V_T, and V_F. These are life-threatening dysrhythmias!

Redrawn from Chernecky, Macklin, Murphy-Ende: *Real-world nursing survival guide: fluids & electrolytes,* Philadelphia, 2001, Saunders, p. 75.

What You DO

When treating patients with hypokalemia, you should remember to do the following:

- Monitor the ECG for ventricular irritability. Potassium replacement therapy may be necessary, particularly if the patient is taking potassium-wasting diuretics.
- Monitor the patient for signs and symptoms of hypokalemia (weakness, fatigue), and teach the patient energy-conserving measures.
- Increase dietary intake of potassium with foods high in potassium, and prescribe supplemental potassium. Foods high in potassium include bananas and dried fruits.
- Administer an antiemetic such as prochlorperazine (Compazine) if hypokalemia is a result of losses through nausea and vomiting; it can be given rectally or by injection.
- Use potassium-sparing diuretics, such as spironolactone (Aldactone), as an alternative to potassium-wasting diuretics, such as Lasix (furosemide).
- Once laboratory results have confirmed a low potassium level, administer potassium either orally or intravenously (IV). It is essential to follow institutional protocols for potassium administration, because potassium given IV can cause vein irritation. It is always diluted when given orally or IV.

TAKE HOME POINTS

Potassium: "No matter the route, always dilute!"

Do You UNDERSTAND?

DIRECTIONS: Fill in the blanks.

1. Name three ways the body can lose potassium.

   _____

   _____

   _____

2. Normal serum potassium level is _____ to _____ mEq/L.

3. An untreated, low potassium can lead to what?

   _____

   _____

   _____

If potassium is given via IV too rapidly, it can cause cardiac arrest.

4. If potassium is administered too rapidly via IV, it can cause what?

   _____

What IS Hyperkalemia?

Hyperkalemia occurs when the serum potassium is greater than 5.2 mEq/L. High levels of potassium cause heart complexes to become wider until they merge into a sine wave. A *sine wave* or *pattern* is a very wide QRS-ST-T pattern that appears as though someone has taken the PQRST and pulled it from the P to the T, trying to pull it apart.

What You NEED TO KNOW

Hyperkalemia can be caused by impaired excretion of potassium as a result of renal disease. Too rapid administration of potassium can cause hyperkalemia. Most of the body's potassium is found inside the cells. Massive tissue injuries, such as crush injuries, myocardial infarction, and burns, can liberate potassium from the cells into the serum.

Laboratory values that reflect a sudden high level of potassium could be the result of poor phlebotomy technique. Using a small needle can destroy red blood cells, causing potassium to be falsely high in the collected specimen. Additionally, removing blood samples from lines that infuse potassium can cause higher levels.

Watch for conditions that cause potassium to shift from the tissues into the bloodstream, such as high-level glucose or acidosis.

Signs and symptoms of hyperkalemia include nausea, vomiting, diarrhea, drowsiness, and mental confusion. Neuromuscular changes, such as weakness or paresthesias, may also occur.

Characteristics of hyperkalemia that are evident on the ECG include small or low-voltage P waves. T waves become very tall and peaked. The monitor may double-count the heart rate if the T becomes as tall as the R wave.

> ⚠ When drawing blood samples from multiple lumen catheters (MLC) or peripheral inserted central catheters (PICCs), the potassium in the IV must be temporarily turned off, and a small sample should be discarded. Otherwise, the patient's potassium may be inappropriately high on the laboratory report, which could lead to inappropriate treatment.
>
> Serum potassium levels should be monitored in patients whose pH is reduced (as caused by respiratory or metabolic acidosis) and in those with increased glucose (as caused by diabetic ketoacidosis).

TAKE HOME POINTS

Hyperkalemia can cause the following ECG changes:
- **Rates and rhythm:** Often a bradycardia or heart block; may result in arrest
- **PR interval:** Small, flattened P waves
- **QRS complex:** Widened
- **QT interval:** Prolonged
- **T waves:** Very tall and peaked
- **Other:** Sine wave or arrest if potassium level is very high

Normal

Hyperkalemia

Sine wave   Sine wave

Redrawn from Chernecky, Macklin, Murphy-Ende: *Real-world nursing survival guide: fluids & electrolytes,* Philadelphia, 2001, Saunders, p. 67.

What You DO

When treating patients with hypokalemia, removing potassium from the serum or driving it back into the cell is the goal. You should remember to do the following:

- Administer non–potassium-sparing diuretics such as furosemide (Lasix) to treat those with mild cases.
- Administer Kayexalate (sodium polystyrene sulfonate) with sorbitol to treat those with moderate cases. Kayexalate binds with potassium in the bowel and eliminates potassium from the body through the feces.
- Administer calcium gluconate to treat those with dangerously high levels of potassium. Calcium gluconate counteracts the negative inotropic effects on the heart.
- Regular insulin and sodium bicarbonate can be added to IVs to drive potassium into the cell when acidosis causes a high level of serum potassium.
- Eliminate all foods, medications, and IVs that contain potassium.
- Consider hemodialysis to decrease serum potassium levels in patients with renal failure or those with severe hyperkalemia.

Do You UNDERSTAND?

DIRECTIONS: **Determine the serum potassium level, ECG signs, and treatment for hypokalemia and hyperkalemia.**

Hypokalemia

1. Serum level: _____

2. ECG signs: _____
   _____
   _____

3. Treatment: _____

Hyperkalemia

4. Serum level: _____

5. ECG signs: _____
   _____

6. Treatment: _____

What IS Hypocalcemia?

Calcium is important for cellular excitability, smooth muscle contractility, and transmission of nerve impulses. Most of the body's calcium is stored in the bone, and only approximately 1% is found in the serum. One half of serum calcium is free or ionized, which is the active form of calcium. The other half is bound to albumin, which is a serum protein.

With normal levels of serum albumin, those with ionized calcium levels below 8.5 mg/dL are considered to have *hypocalcemia*. Calcium is needed by the cardiac cells to help with contraction. When calcium is low, the heart does not beat as strongly as it should.

Answers: **1. Less than 3.5mEq/L;** 2. prolonged PR intervals; U wave, PVCs can lead to ventricular tachycardia; 3. K⁺ replacement oral or Iv; 4. greater than 5.2 mEq/L; 5. small P wave, tall peaked T wave, prolonged QRS, bradycardias, cardiac arrest; 6. diuretics, calcium, HCO_3, and insulin, Kayexalate, hemodialysis.

What You NEED TO KNOW

Causes of low calcium include hypomagnesemia or hypoparathyroidism. A decreased dietary intake of calcium, as well as diarrhea, can cause calcium loss. Because one half of the serum calcium is bound to serum proteins (albumin), a low level of blood proteins will also lower the level of serum calcium. Prolonged bedrest with limited vitamin D and exposure to sunlight can cause hypocalcemia in critically or chronically ill patients. Surgical removal of the parathyroid can also result in hypocalcemia. As the level of serum phosphorus increases, calcium decreases. Calcium can be lost in burn fluid, peritonitis, and infection. A calcium below 8.5 mg/dL can cause the QT interval to prolong. The T waves may become flatter. A low serum calcium level can cause ventricular dysrhythmias.

TAKE HOME POINTS

Magnesium and calcium deficiencies are often found together. Monitor the magnesium level as well.

Normal	Hypocalcemia

TAKE HOME POINTS

Hypocalcemia on a 12-lead ECG can cause the following changes:
- **Rate:** May be anything
- **Rhythm:** Possible regular, ventricular dysrhythmias
- **PR interval:** Can be prolonged
- **QRS complex:** Lengthened
- **ST segment and T wave:** Flattened
- **QT interval:** Prolonged

What You DO

When treating patients with hypocalcemia, you should remember to do the following:
- Observe and monitor calcium levels and report any abnormal levels to the health care provider.
- Assess the patient for signs and symptoms of a low level of calcium. Chvostek's sign (facial twitching after a finger tap on the supramandibular portion of the parotid gland) and Trousseau's sign (carpopedal spasm

after inflation of blood pressure cuff to upper arm) are indicators of the neuromuscular irritability that accompanies hypocalcemia.

- Be prepared for emergency airway management, which may include endotracheal intubation or tracheostomy. Patients with low levels of calcium can have laryngeal spasms, resulting in airway obstruction.

 The patient may exhibit signs or symptoms of decreased cardiac contractility. Cardiovascular effects can include decreased cardiac output and congestive heart failure, which can lead to cardiac arrest.

Do You UNDERSTAND?

DIRECTIONS: Provide answers to the following questions.

1. Hypocalcemia may have what electrophysiologic effects?

_____

_____

_____

2. What neuromuscular signs does hypocalcemia include?

_____

_____

_____

_____

_____

3. A true medical emergency of hypocalcemia includes what? *(Give at least two symptoms.)*

_____

_____

_____

_____

 TAKE HOME POINTS

Low levels of calcium are treated with the oral administration of calcium, IV push, or IV infusion of calcium gluconate chloride.

What IS Hypercalcemia?

Hypercalcemia is a calcium blood level of above 11 mg/dL. High levels of calcium affect the heart by reducing threshold potential and decreasing excitability.

What You NEED TO KNOW

Hypercalcemia is caused by excessive bone reabsorption of calcium, which is often the result of an increase in parathyroid hormone or metastatic cancers. The body usually increases renal excretion of calcium when there is either greater dietary consumption or ingestion of calcium supplements. Hypercalcemia can also occur if there is ingestion of increased calcium in the presence of kidney failure.

ECG changes from hypercalcemia may include a shortened ST segment and QT interval and a prolonged PR interval and QRS complex. In severe hypercalcemia, AV blocks may occur.

TAKE HOME POINTS

High calcium can cause the following ECG changes:
* **Rate:** Slow
* **Rhythm:** May be variable
* **PR interval:** Normal
* **QRS complex:** Progressive widening
* **QT segment:** Shortened

Normal	Hypercalcemia

Women who are taking calcium supplements to prevent the effects of osteoporosis should be taught the correct dose and the importance of hydration to prevent the formation of kidney stones.

What You DO

When treating patients with hypercalcemia, you should remember to do the following:
* Monitor calcium levels and the neurologic status of the patient. Fatigue, loss of deep tendon reflexes (DTRs), thirst, constipation, and kidney stones may be present.
* Administer large amounts of IV saline to dilute the calcium and help it pass from the body.

- Administer loop diuretics, if prescribed.
- Administer IV phosphate, if prescribed. Phosphate and calcium work in opposition. As the phosphate levels rise, calcium levels decrease.
- Eliminate foods containing calcium from the patient's diet.
- Include cytotoxic antibiotics (e.g., Mithracin) and hormones (e.g., calcitonin) that block bone release of calcium as a treatment of extreme hypercalcemia.

Do You UNDERSTAND?

DIRECTIONS: **Complete the following exercises.**

1. List four risks for hypercalcemia.

    _____

    _____

    _____

    _____

2. Describe three ECG changes observed with hypercalcemia.

    _____

    _____

    _____

What IS Hypomagnesemia?

Magnesium is primarily found in the cells and bones. It is important for maintaining neuromuscular activities, blood clotting, and normal cardiac-action potentials. A low level of magnesium places patients at risk for developing a lethal form of VT, known as torsades de pointes. *Hypomagnesemia* is a condition in which the magnesium level falls below 1.5 mEq/L.

A decrease in the level of magnesium slows the release of an enzyme called acetylcholine. Acetylcholine helps stimulate the parasympathetic nervous system. Therefore a low level of magnesium will increase the fight-or-flight response.

Answers: 1. prolonged bedrest, renal failure, hyperparathyroidism, patients with cancer may be at risk for hypercalcemia; 2. short or absent ST segment, decreased QT interval, prolonged PR and QRS.

What You NEED TO KNOW

A low level of magnesium has the same effects as hypocalcemia, and it has the same causes. Review the discussion of hypocalcemia in this chapter.

What You DO

When administering magnesium sulfate, the patient's heart rate, blood pressure, respirations, Sao$_2$, ECG, and neurologic changes must be monitored. Deep tendon reflexes and the level of consciousness must be evaluated, because an increased magnesium can also lead to cardiac arrest as a result of inadequate heart stimulation.

When treating patients with hypomagnesemia, you should remember to do the following:
• Identify low levels of magnesium and determine the causes.
• Assess for signs of neuromuscular irritability and institute seizure precautions.
• Consider prescribing calcium or magnesium supplements. Magnesium sulfate may be given as a continuous or intermittent infusion. A typical dose is 2 to 6 g IV over several minutes.
• Watch for potassium depletion, which may also occur with hypomagnesemia.

Do You UNDERSTAND?

DIRECTIONS: **Indicate in the spaces provided whether the following statements are *true* or *false*.**
1. _____ Dose is 3.5 to 5.2 mEq/kg.
2. _____ Dose is always given diluted.
3. _____ Dose is 2 to 6 g IV push.
4. _____ Calcium supplements may also be given.
5. _____ Can be mixed in an IV bag and administered via drip.

Answers: **1. False; 2. False; 3. True; 4. True; 5. True.**

What IS Hypermagnesemia?

Magnesium is a cell membrane stabilizer. *Hypermagnesemia* is an elevated level of magnesium, and it causes the cells to be less sensitive to stimuli. If the levels are high, the cells may not respond to *any* stimulus. The clinical presentation of a high level of magnesium includes muscle weakness, confusion, and respiratory paralysis. At levels greater than 6 mEq/L, the patient may develop bradycardia, hypotension, increased PR intervals, widened QRS complexes, and elevated T waves.

A high level of magnesium is similar to a high level of calcium. Review the section on hypercalcemia in the chapter.

What You NEED TO KNOW

High levels of magnesium can be caused by increases in the rate of IV solutions that contain magnesium, such as parenteral nutrition or hyper-alimentation solutions. Antacids that contain magnesium include aluminum hydroxide (Maalox) and simethicone (Mylanta). Overuse of antacids can cause the magnesium levels to rise. In addition, overuse of laxatives such as magnesium hydroxide (Milk of Magnesia) can cause hypermagnesemia.

What You DO

When treating patients with hypercalcemia, you should remember to do the following:
- Monitor serum magnesium levels.
- Observe for the early signs of hypermagnesemia.
- Assess the use of over-the-counter medications for the potential effects of hypermagnesemia.
- If prescribed, administer calcium gluconate to treat the cardiac effects of hypermagnesemia.
- If prescribed, administer diuretics to increase magnesium loss.
- Monitor vital signs and cardiac status.

 Diuretics should be administered only to patients with normal renal function.

Do You UNDERSTAND?

⚠ Observe the patient for signs of respiratory depression. Resuscitation equipment should be readily available.

DIRECTIONS: **Place a check next to the features associated with hyper-magnesemia.**

1. _____ Magnesium level < 1.5 mEq/L
2. _____ Magnesium level > 2 mEq/L
3. _____ Shortened QT interval
4. _____ Administer magnesium sulfate
5. _____ Administer diuretics/saline infusions

References

Aehlert B: *ECGs made easy,* ed 2, St Louis, 2002, Mosby.

American Heart Association: *Advanced cardiac life support provider manual,* Dallas, 1997, American Heart Association.

Anderson K, editor: *Mosby's medical, nursing and allied health dictionary,* ed 5, St Louis, 1998, Mosby.

Chernecky C, Berger B: *Laboratory tests and diagnostic procedures,* ed 4, Philadelphia, 2004, Saunders.

Copstead LEC, Banasik JC: *Pathophysiology: biological and behavioral perspectives,* ed 2, Philadelphia, 2000, Saunders.

Davenport J, Morton PG: Identifying nonischemic causes of life-threatening arrhythmias, *Am J Nurs* 97(11):50, 1997.

Ehrat K: *The art of EKG interpretation: a self-instructional text,* ed 4, Dubuque, IA, 1997, Kendall Hunt.

Lamborn ML, Moseley MJ: Cardiac alterations. In Hartshorn JC, Sole ML, Lamborn ML, editors: *Introduction to critical care nursing,* ed 3, Philadelphia, 2001, Saunders.

McCoy C, Livingston N: Cardiovascular laboratory and diagnostic tests. In Bucher L, Melander S: *Critical care nursing,* Philadelphia, 1999, Saunders.

Skidmore L: *Mosby's drug guide for nurses,* St Louis, 2001, Mosby.

Thelan LA et al: *Critical care nursing: diagnosis and management,* ed 3, St Louis, 1998, Mosby.

Answers: 2, 3, 5.

NCLEX® Review

1. ECG changes indicative of hyperkalemia include:
   1 Prolonged QT intervals
   2 ST-segment depression
   3 Tall, peaked T waves
   4 Decreased T-wave amplitude

2. Digitalis may have all of the following effects on the ECG except to:
   1 Shorten the QT interval
   2 Prolong the PR interval
   3 Cause scooping of the ST segments
   4 Increase the heart rate

3. Calcium channel blockers may be used for all of the following except:
   1 Supraventricular tachycardias
   2 Heart blocks
   3 Atrial tachycardias
   4 Hypertension

4. ECG changes indicating hypokalemia may include:
   1 ST-segment depression
   2 Prolonged QT intervals
   3 Development of U waves
   4 Tall, peaked T waves

5. Class IA antidysrhythmics include all of the following except:
   1 Lidocaine hydrochloride
   2 Quinidine sulfate
   3 Disopyramide (Norpace)
   4 Procainamide (Pronestyl)

6. Scooping of the ST segment, heart blocks, bradycardia, and prolonged PR intervals are all characteristics of _____ toxicity.
   1 Digitalis (Lanoxin)
   2 Potassium
   3 Procainamide (Pronestyl)
   4 Quinidine (Quinaglute)

7. The patient's potassium level is 3.2 mEq/L. The health care provider knows replacement of potassium is:
   1 Done by administering a 20 mEq potassium bolus
   2 Always done with the potassium diluted
   3 Always done with intramuscular injections
   4 Usually given via rectal suppository

8. The most frequent cause of hypokalemia in a patient is _____ therapy.
   1 Corticosteroid
   2 Diuretic
   3 Calcium
   4 Digoxin

NCLEX® Review Answers

1. 3 Tall, peaked T waves may occur with hyperkalemia. Prolonged QT intervals, ST-segment depression, and decreased T-wave amplitude are all signs of hypokalemia.

2. 4 Digitalis typically decreases the heart rate. Digitalis may also shorten the QT interval and prolong the PR interval. A hallmark sign of digitalis effect is ST-segment scooping.

3. 2 Calcium channel blockers should never be given to patients with bradycardia, sick sinus syndrome, or heart blocks. Calcium channel blockers are used to treat supraventricular tachycardias because they slow atrioventricular conduction time and increase the refractoriness of the atrioventricular node. Calcium channel blockers may be used for patients with atrial tachycardias because they slow atrioventricular conduction time. Calcium channel blockers lower blood pressure and can be used in cases of hypertension.

4. **4** Hyperkalemia results in tall, peaked T waves. ST-segment depression, prolonged QT intervals, and the occurrence of U waves indicate hypokalemia.

5. **1** Lidocaine is considered a class IB agent. Quinidine, disopyramide, and procainamide are class IA agents. Class IA agents slow the influx of sodium into the cardiac cell and decrease the rate of depolarization.

6. **1** Scooping of the ST segments, heart blocks, bradycardia, and prolonging of PR intervals are the ECG signs of digitoxicity. Potassium changes depend on whether the patient is hypokalemic or hyperkalemic. ECG changes characteristic of class IA antidysrhythmics include long PR intervals, QRS, and QT. Quinidine and procainamide are class IA antidysrhythmic drugs.

7. **2** No matter the route, potassium is always diluted. Potassium given by rapid IV bolus can result in ventricular fibrillation and death. Potassium is never given by the intramuscular route because it irritates the tissues. Potassium is not readily absorbed as a rectal suppository and is also very irritating to those tissues.

8. **2** Most loop diuretics cause potassium wasting. Corticosteroids cause water retention and hyponatremia. There is no correlation between calcium excess and potassium depletion. Combination therapy of loop diuretic and cardiac glycoside (digoxin) causes hypokalemia.

Conduction Defects and Accessory Pathways

What You WILL LEARN

After reading this chapter, you will know how to do the following:
- ✔ Define LGL syndrome.
- ✔ State one patient condition associated with LGL syndrome.
- ✔ Define WPW syndrome.
- ✔ State one patient condition associated with WPW syndrome.

This chapter covers special conduction syndromes that may occur in your patients. Two of the more common conduction system defects, (1) Lown-Ganong-Levine (LGL) syndrome and (2) Wolff-Parkinson-White (WPW) syndrome, and the accessory pathways associated with them are discussed.

What IS LGL Syndrome?

LGL syndrome is a rhythm caused by the presence of an alternative conduction pathway that bridges the atria and ventricles by avoiding the atrioventricular (AV) node and entering the upper end of the bundle of His. The accessory pathway is referred to as James fibers.

This disorder was first described by the American physicians Lown and Levine and by physiologist Ganong. It is characterized by a stimulus bypassing the atrioventricular (AV) node and exciting the ventricles earlier than normal. Patients with this syndrome, which is difficult to detect, may complain of intermittent palpitations and experience supraventricular tachydysrhythmias.

What You NEED TO KNOW

When a stimulus bypasses the AV node in LGL, the PR interval is shortened, because the impulse is not delayed at the AV node. There is no pre-excitation of the ventricular muscle; therefore there is no aberrant ventricular conduction. For this reason, LGL syndrome is sometimes called the short PR normal QRS syndrome.

Redrawn from Paul, Hebra: *The nurse's guide to cardiac rhythm interpretation,* Philadelphia, 1998, Saunders, p. 252.

Supraventricular tachycardia (SVT) is also one of the distinguishing features of LGL syndrome. The tachycardias in LGL syndrome are thought to be from an AV-reciprocating mechanism that causes a marked difference in conduction times between retrograde conduction up the fast (bypass) pathway and slow conduction down the regular nodal pathway, providing opportunity for reentry (reactivation of a tissue for the second time by the same impulse).

What IS WPW Syndrome?

WPW syndrome is an abnormal condition in which the ventricles are stimulated by an early impulse traveling down an alternative conduction pathway that bridges the atria and ventricles either anteriorly or posteriorly. This conduction pathway is called *Kent's bundle.* Because of the presence of Kent's bundle, descending atrial impulses have two routes between the atria and ventricles. The accessory pathway has a greater conduction velocity than the normal conduction pathway because it bypasses the delay at the AV node.

What You NEED TO KNOW

In WPW syndrome, a depolarization wave from the sinoatrial (SA) node may reach the AV node and the accessory pathway at the same time; the impulses traversing the two pathways may reach the ventricular cells at different times.

The characteristics of WPW syndrome include the following:

- PR interval is short (less than 0.12 seconds). Unlike the PR interval in LGL syndrome, the PR interval in WPW syndrome has a delta wave. A delta wave is a slurring of the QRS complex, resulting from impulses traveling to the ventricles by different conduction pathways and depolarizing the ventricular myocardium from different directions at the same time.
- QRS complex is 0.12 seconds wide or wider. Aberrant ventricular conduction is present.
- Rate can be normal or fast. Patients with WPW may experience dysrhythmias, such as supraventricular (SVT), atrial flutter, and atrial fibrillation. Supraventricular tachydysrhythmias in WPW may result from a reentry circuit using the accessory pathway and the AV node. If the patient develops atrial fibrillation, the ventricular rate may become so rapid that the rhythm will deteriorate to ventricular fibrillation.
- Patients with WPW may or may not have symptoms.
- In WPW patients, the onset of atrial fibrillation promotes the risk for rapid ventricular response through the accessory pathway causing the clinical manifestations of stable and unstable tachycardias.

TAKE HOME POINTS

The characteristics of LGL syndrome include the following:
- **PR interval:** Short (less than 0.12 seconds)
- **QRS complex:** Normal width (less than 0.12 seconds)
- **Rhythms:** Fast supraventricular rhythms
- **Other:** Holter monitoring may be used for 24-hour observation

TAKE HOME POINTS

The characteristics of WPW syndrome include the following:
- **PR interval:** Short (less than 0.12 seconds).
- **QRS complex:** Aberrant ventricular conduction; 0.12 seconds wide or wider
- **Rate:** Normal or fast

Redrawn from Paul, Hebra: *The nurse's guide to cardiac rhythm interpretation,* Philadelphia, 1998, Saunders, p. 244.

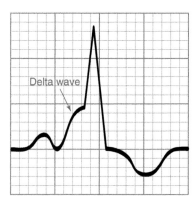

Redrawn from Paul, Hebra: *The nurse's guide to cardiac rhythm interpretation,* Philadelphia, 1998, Saunders, p. 244.

What You DO

The treatments for LGL and WPW are very similar. In patients with LGL, electrical physiologic studies (EPSs) may be performed to determine the location of the abnormal conduction pathway. EPSs are invasive tests that determine more about the abnormal conduction in the heart and the specific, effective therapy for the conduction disturbance.

Surgical interruption or radio frequency ablation of the abnormal AV pathway may be indicated in patients with LGL syndrome. Complications of radio frequency ablation may include postprocedure heart blocks.

If either LGL or WPW is apparent, observe for fast, tachydysrhythmias. Based on ACLS guidelines, focus evaluation of the patient on the following:

- Is the patient clinically unstable? (Experiencing symptoms such as hypotension, chest pain, shortness of breath, or any change in level of consciousness)
- Does the patient have impaired cardiac function? (Based on echocardiogram that shows an ejection fraction < 40%).
- Is WPW present?
- Is the duration of the tachycardia ≤ or ≥ 48 hours?
  The treatment is focused on the following:
- Treat unstable patients urgently.
- Control the ventricular rate.
- Ensure that atrial fibrillation or flutter is not present. In a normal heart, cardioversion or antidysrhythmic therapy such as amiodarone, flecainide, or procainamide can be used. In an impaired heart (ejection fraction < 40%), cardioversion or amiodarone should be used.
- Convert the rhythm.
- If the duration of the WPW tachycardia is ≤ 48 hours, cardioversion or antiarrhythmics such as amiodarone, flecainide, or procainamide can be used. If the ejection fraction is diminished impaired cardiac function, cardioversion or amiodarone should be used.
- Provide anticoagulation. If the duration is > 48 hours, the patient should be anticoagulated for 3 weeks prior to cardioversion and anticoagulated for an additional 4 weeks postcardioversion.
- Overdrive pacing may be successful in terminating the rhythm.

> ⚠️ Drugs that can be harmful in treating atrial fibrillation with WPW include adenosine, α blockers, calcium channel blockers, and digoxin.

Do You UNDERSTAND?

DIRECTIONS: **Fill in the blanks.**

1. List three characteristics of LGL syndrome.

   _____

   _____

   _____

DIRECTIONS: **Place a check in the spaces under each conduction syndrome (LGL or WPW) if the symptom is associated with the syndrome(s).**

	LGL	WPW	Symptom
2.	_____	_____	Short PR interval
3.	_____	_____	Long QRS
4.	_____	_____	Delta wave
5.	_____	_____	Normal QRS
6.	_____	_____	Tachydysrythmias
7.	_____	_____	Long QT interval

DIRECTIONS: **Fill in the blanks.**

8. In a patient who has WPW or LGL syndrome with a tachycardia, the clinical evaluation should be focused on the following:

_____

_____

_____

_____

9. The treatment focus should be based on:

_____

_____

_____

_____

10. Drugs that can be harmful in treating patients with atrial fibrillation with WPW syndrome are:

_____

_____

_____

_____

DIRECTIONS: **Complete the crossword puzzle.**

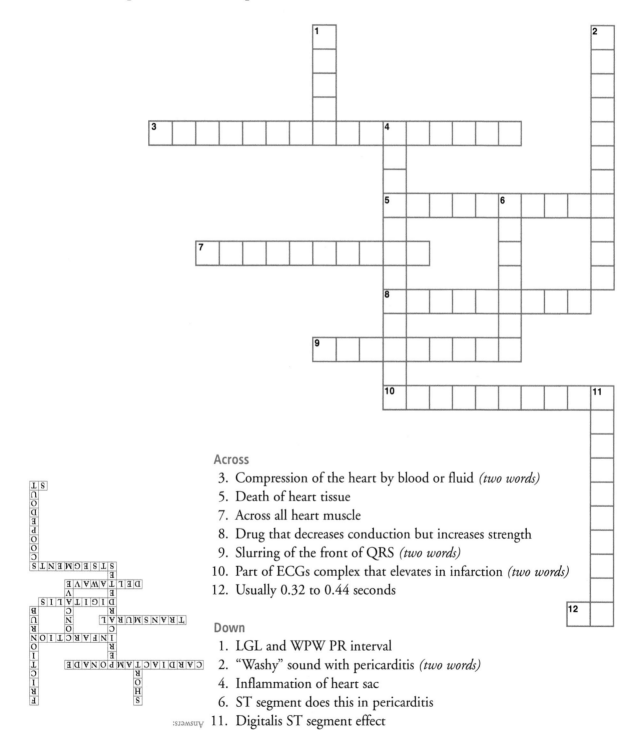

Across

3. Compression of the heart by blood or fluid *(two words)*
5. Death of heart tissue
7. Across all heart muscle
8. Drug that decreases conduction but increases strength
9. Slurring of the front of QRS *(two words)*
10. Part of ECGs complex that elevates in infarction *(two words)*
12. Usually 0.32 to 0.44 seconds

Down

1. LGL and WPW PR interval
2. "Washy" sound with pericarditis *(two words)*
4. Inflammation of heart sac
6. ST segment does this in pericarditis
11. Digitalis ST segment effect

Answers:

References

Aehlert B: *ECGs made easy,* ed 2, St Louis, 2002, Mosby.

American Heart Association: *Advanced cardiac life support provider manual,* Dallas, 1997, American Heart Association.

Anderson K: *Mosby's medical, nursing, and allied health dictionary,* ed 5, St Louis, 1998, Mosby.

Conover MB: *Understanding electrocardiography,* ed 5, St Louis, 1988, Mosby.

Copstead LEC, Banasik JC: *Pathophysiology: biological and behavioral perspectives,* ed 2, Philadelphia, 2000, Saunders.

Cummins RO: *Advanced cardiac life support,* Dallas, 1997, American Heart Association.

Davenport J, Morton PG: Identifying nonischemic causes of life-threatening arrhythmias, *Am J Nurs* 97(11):50, 1997.

Dugan K: Caring for patients with pericarditis, *Nursing* 28(3):50, 1998.

Ehrat K: *The art of EKG interpretation: a self-instructional text,* ed 4, Dubuque, IA, 1997, Kendall Hunt.

Grauer K: *A practical guide to ECG interpretation,* St Louis, 1992, Mosby.

Huszar R: *Basic dysrhythmias: interpretation and management,* ed 2, St Louis, 1994, Mosby.

Kotecki CN: Infectious cardiac disorders. In Bucher L, Melander S: *Critical care nursing,* Philadelphia, 1999, Saunders.

Kupper NS, Duke ES: Inflammatory and valvular heart disease. In Lewis SM, Heitkemper MM, Dirksen SR: *Medical surgical nursing: assessment and management of clinical problems,* ed 5, St Louis, 2000, Mosby.

Lamborn ML, Moseley MJ: Cardiac alterations. In Hartshorn JC, Sole ML, Lamborn ML, editors: *Introduction to critical care nursing,* ed 3, Philadelphia, 2001, Saunders.

Lazzara D, Sellergren C: Chest pain: making the right call when the pressure is on, *Nursing 96* 26(11):42, 1996.

Makrevis C: Understanding non-Q wave MI, *Nursing 94* 24(8):32CC, 1994.

McCoy C, Livingston N: Cardiovascular laboratory and diagnostic tests. In Bucher L, Melander S: *Critical care nursing,* Philadelphia, 1999, Saunders.

Pierce CO: Acute post-MI pericarditis, *J Cardiovasc Nurs* 6(4):46, 1992.

Sims JM, Miracle V: Using the ECG to detect myocardial infarction. *Nursing* 29(8):41, 1999.

Skidmore L: *Mosby's drug guide for nurses,* St Louis, 2001, Mosby.

Thelan LA et al: *Critical Care nursing: diagnosis and management,* ed 3, St Louis, 1998, Mosby.

Wharton JM, Goldschlager N: *Guide to interpreting 12-lead ECGs,* Oradell, NJ, 1984, Medical Economics Books.

NCLEX® Review

1. A condition that may contribute to rapid heart rates and that is characterized by an accessory pathway called the bundle of Kent is:
   1 Atrial fibrillation
   2 Wolff-Parkinson-White (WPW) syndrome
   3 Lown-Ganong-Levine (LGL) syndrome
   4 Complete heart block

2. Which of the following is not a characteristic of LGL syndrome?
   1 Short PR interval
   2 Normal width QRS complex
   3 Delta wave
   4 Supraventricular tachycardias

3. Which of the following is NOT a characteristic of WPW syndrome?
   1 Short PR interval
   2 Aberrant ventricular conduction
   3 Delta wave
   4 Normal width QRS complex

4. In LGL syndrome, what is the accessory pathway called?

5. What is premature activation of the ventricular myocardium referred to as?

NCLEX® Review Answers

1. 2 The accessory pathway in WPW syndrome is the bundle of Kent. Atrial fibrillation does not have an accessory pathway via bundle of Kent, LGL bypasses the AV node through James fibers, and complete heart block is not characterized by tachycardia.

2. 3 In LGL syndrome, there is preexcitation because the impulse bypasses the atrioventricular node by way of James fibers. Because there is no conduction through the atrioventricular node, there is no potential for a delta wave to occur. A short PR interval, a normal width QRS complex, and supraventricular tachycardias are all characteristics of LGL syndrome.

3. 4 Aberrant ventricular contraction occurs because the ventricles are stimulated by the bundle of Kent and via the atrioventricular node, causing a wide QRS complex. A short PR interval, aberrant ventricular conduction, and a delta wave are characteristics of WPW syndrome.

4. The accessory pathway in LGL syndrome is James fibers.

5. Preexcitation is activation of the ventricular myocardium sooner than normal.

Notes

Special Considerations

What You WILL LEARN

After reading this chapter, you will know how to do the following:
- ✔ Explain the purpose of an ICD.
- ✔ State the purpose of a pacemaker.
- ✔ Explain the purpose of coronary artery bypass grafting.
- ✔ Define cardiac transplantation.
- ✔ State two conditions that would warrant cardiac transplant.
- ✔ Describe cardiac trauma.
- ✔ List two possible causes of cardiac trauma.
- ✔ List two possible sequelae associated with cardiac trauma.

This chapter provides a synopsis of major cardiac events that have special considerations for electrocardiogram (ECG) monitoring. Four distinct areas provide reference for ECG considerations pertaining to electrical cardiac therapy, drug abuse, surgical therapy, and cardiac trauma.

ELECTRICAL CARDIAC THERAPY

Sudden cardiac death (SCD) is a syndrome in which the heart abruptly stops beating. Most SCD episodes occur when the irritable, diseased heart impulses become too rapid as in ventricular tachycardia or chaotic as in ventricular fibrillation. The result is that the heart is unable to pump blood, and brain death will occur within minutes if left untreated. SCD can be reversed but treatment must take place almost immediately following the arrest. Because SCD is related to ventricular fibrillation (VF) in most adults, early cardiopulmonary resuscitation (CPR) and defibrillation are required to return the heart rhythm to normal. For patients with significant risk for SCD, an **implantable cardioverter-defibrillator (ICD)** may be inserted as a preventive measure.

What IS an ICD?

An *ICD* is a device that continuously monitors the heart rate and rhythm. It is designed to detect and treat life-threatening dysrhythmias, such as ventricular tachycardia (VT) and ventricular fibrillation (VF). It is also used to treat less-threatening conditions, such as atrial fibrillation. When a dangerous rhythm is recognized, the ICD provides a shock (**electrical stimulation**) directly to the heart muscle to stop the dysrhythmia and allow the heart to resume its normal electrical pattern. The device consists of one or more thin, insulated wires (**leads**) that are in contact with the heart muscle and connected to an implanted pulse generator. Rapid technologic advancements in electrophysiology have produced sophisticated ICDs that can be programmed to deliver a variety of patterns and intensities of electrical therapy in response to abnormal rhythms. The sensation experienced by the individual when the device discharges varies with the pattern and intensity of the therapy. The shock may be felt as tingling or it may be painful. In some instances, an individual may be conscious and not even be aware that the device has discharged.

Electromagnetic interference from electronic antitheft surveillance devices (often used in stores and libraries) can cause circuitry failure. Should this happen, you should move the patient away from the antitheft equipment immediately.

Transcutaneous nerve stimulators (TENS) used for pain control can create electrical artifact, leading to inappropriate ICD delivery.

What You NEED TO KNOW

ICDs use electrical impulses to control life-threatening dysrhythmias. These devices are programmed to recognize certain rhythms and deliver specified electrical therapy. ICDs are implanted in a procedure very similar to pacemaker implantation. The surgeon guides the lead placement through a major vein via fluoroscopy, and the generator is implanted in a superficial skin pocket in the abdomen or upper chest. There is a small

Magnet mode is very important during acute resuscitation efforts, because the functioning of the ICD may interfere with emergency treatment.

Do not use a TENS (transcutaneous electrical nerve stimulation) unit on someone with an ICD, because it will create artifact leading to ICD delivery.

risk of infection with the procedure. A standard pacemaker magnet placed over the ICD pulse generator activates the *magnet mode* feature. Although the magnet mode feature varies among manufacturers; it is generally used to *suppress* ICD therapy.

Symptoms of a malfunctioning ICD may include the following:
- Dizziness
- Syncope
- Palpitations
- Inappropriate "shocks"

If you suspect that a patient's ICD is malfunctioning, you must continuously monitor the electrocardiograph (ECG) for VT or VF.

Most household electrical devices do not interfere with ICD function. Strong electrical and magnetic fields (including those used in magnetic resonance imaging [MRI]) have the potential to interfere with the sensing circuitry of ICDs. Electromagnetic security systems found in high security areas such as airports and courthouses should be avoided or the patient with an ICD simply move through them at a normal pace, avoiding the device, if possible, and certainly avoiding leaning on or touching it.

What You DO

When treating patients with ICDs, you should remember the following:
- During the admission assessment, obtain as much information as possible regarding the device used by the patient. Ask if the patient was given an "ICD information and identification card" when the device was implanted. If no card is available, determine the approximate date of implantation. Generally, newer devices are more sophisticated than those implanted years ago.
- Keep resuscitation equipment handy if the device is suspected of malfunctioning.
- Continuously monitor the ECG of a symptomatic patient. Watch for signs of VT and VF.
- Have a pacemaker magnet available to deactivate the ICD if necessary.
- If you are unfamiliar with the functions of the particular device, call for assistance before placing a magnet near the ICD generator.

- If dangerous rhythms (VT, VF) occur despite the presence of an ICD, resuscitate the patient per Advanced Cardiac Life Support (ACLS) guidelines.
- Advise patients to stay away from strong magnetic fields, as in MRIs.

ECG Findings in VT

- **Rate:** Rapid ventricular rate greater than 100 beats/min; usually 200 to 300 beats/min
- **Rhythm:** Usually not possible to determine the atrial rhythm; regular ventricular rhythm
- **P waves:** Usually not visible; obscured by the QRS complexes
- **QRS complex:** Wide (greater than 0.12 seconds)

TAKE HOME POINTS

Cellular telephones only interfere with ICDs during telemetric transmission and programming. Otherwise they are safe for use by patients with ICDs.

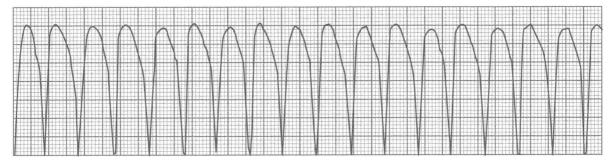

Redrawn from Cohn, Gilroy-Doohan: *Flip and see ECG,* Philadelphia, 1996, Saunders, p. 91.

ECG Findings in VF

- **Rate:** Not measurable
- **Rhythm:** Irregular, chaotic
- **P waves:** Not visible
- **QRS complex:** No identifiable complexes

VF is rapidly fatal if left untreated.

Redrawn from Cohn, Gilroy-Doohan: *Flip and see ECG,* Philadelphia, 1996, Saunders, p. 91.

Do You UNDERSTAND?

DIRECTIONS: **Indicate in the spaces provided whether the following statements are *true* or *false*.**

1. _____ ICD devices are one of the **initial** techniques used to treat rhythm disturbances.
2. _____ ICDs detect potentially lethal dysrhythmias.
3. _____ Placement of an ICD requires an open thoracostomy procedure.
4. _____ A patient who has a potentially lethal arrhythmia despite the presence of an ICD should be resuscitated according to ACLS guidelines.
5. _____ The ICD device consists of one or more insulated metal leads in contact with the myocardial tissue and connected to a pulse generator.

DIRECTIONS: **Unscramble the letters in the word jumble to fill in the blanks. When all words in the jumble have been unscrambled and entered into the blanks, the circled letters form one last jumbled word. What is it?**

6. __ ◯ ◯ __ __ __ __ SIPLUME

7. __ __ ◯ __ __ __ __ __ __ __ __ VERANTUSSNO

8. __ ◯ __ ◯ __ ◯ __ __ __ TEERGARON

9. __ __ __ ◯ __ ◯ __ __ __ __ LETILCAER

10. __ __ __ __ ◯ OKCHS

11. ◯◯◯◯◯◯◯◯◯ CAEPMKRAE

DIRECTIONS: **Answer the following questions.**

12. What potential danger could occur if a patient with an ICD stands near the generator of a department store's alarm system?

13. Your patient has an ICD and asks you if he or she can use his cellular telephone. What is your response?

What IS a Pacemaker?

Heart muscle contracts when it is stimulated by an electrical impulse. This electrical impulse normally originates in the sinoatrial (SA) node of the right ventricle and travels along a specific pathway to the ventricles. This specialized function has earned the SA node the title of "the heart's natural pacemaker." Deviations from the usual electrical impulse pattern cause changes in heart rhythm. The heart may beat too fast or slow. Perhaps the designated pathway is blocked, preventing impulses from reaching their destination. When the heart's natural pacemaker falters, an artificial pacemaker can be inserted to restore a healthy electrical impulse pattern.

A *pacemaker* is a programmable, battery-operated device that delivers a precisely timed electrical impulse to the heart muscle. The electrical impulse comes from the pacemaker generator and is delivered through thin insulated wires called *leads*. The electrical stimulus is seen on the ECG as a pacemaker *spike*. If depolarization occurs, it will be observed as a P wave (atrial depolarization) or QRS complex (ventricular depolarization). The term *capture* indicates that the electrical stimulus has successfully depolarized the heart muscle and now controls the chamber.

Most pacemakers *sense* the heart's naturally occurring rhythm and deliver the battery-generated impulse only when the intrinsic rate falls below a preset limit; this is called *demand pacing*. In certain emergency situations (when a patient is asystolic or extremely bradycardic), *fixed rate pacing* delivers the electrical stimulus, regardless of the patient's own heart rhythm.

Answers: **12. The patient may experience pacemaker circuitry failure; 13. The patient can use the cellular phone, but not during telemetric transmission or ICD programming.**

Pacer spike with capture. (Redrawn from Ignatavicius, Workman, Mishler: *Medical-surgical nursing across the health care continuum,* ed 2, Philadelphia, 1995, Saunders, p. 792.)

Temporary Versus Permanent Pacemakers

Temporary pacemakers are used in emergency situations and for short-term therapy. Leads for a temporary pacing system may be placed directly into the heart muscle during cardiac surgery and exit through the skin of the chest wall (**epicardial leads**). This type of pacing commonly occurs with postoperative cardiac surgery patients. Temporary leads might also be threaded into place through a large vein via a central venous catheter; this is called transvenous pacing. The temporary leads for both epicardial and transvenous pacing are attached to a generator box that remains outside the body where the settings are adjusted manually. Exposed transvenous or epicardial pacing wires should be insulated to prevent delivery of unintentional *microshocks* to the heart muscle. Because the wires are in direct contact with the heart muscle, even weak static-generated electrical impulses can be problematic. In emergency situations, temporary pacing is sometimes accomplished via electrode patches placed on the chest wall. This is called *transcutaneous pacing* and is used until a temporary or a permanent pacer can be inserted.

Leads for a *permanent pacemaker* are usually guided to the inner heart wall through a large vein using radiographic images (**fluoroscopy** or **transvenous placement**). The leads are tunneled beneath the skin, connecting the heart muscle to the pacemaker. Permanent pacemakers are about the size of a silver dollar and weigh approximately 1 ounce.

Modern, implanted permanent pacemakers are true wonders of technology. The feature that makes them so useful in the treatment of dysrhythmias is their ability to be *programmed* transdermally to meet the needs of the individual. The programmer is a device that uses radio waves to communicate with the pacemaker's pulse generator. The pacemaker generator can be reprogrammed without surgery because the radio frequencies are detected through the skin.

Pacemaker *check-ups* can take place over the telephone. Information about the individual's rhythm, the status of the pulse generator's battery, and the pacemaker's pacing capability are delivered to the medical facility by a transmitting unit over telephone lines.

What You NEED TO KNOW

Troubleshooting a dual-chamber pacemaker may be difficult, especially if you are unsure how it is programmed. The general rule is to notify the primary health care provider if the patient is symptomatic or there is any suggestion of pacer malfunction. Symptoms of *malfunctioning* pacemaker may include the following:
• Dizziness
• Fainting spells (syncope)
• Change in mental status
• Difficulty breathing
• Prolonged weakness or fatigue
• Prolonged hiccups
  Vital signs may reveal the following:
• Decreased heart rate (less than preset low limit)
• Increased heart rate (greater than 100 bpm)
• Irregular heart rhythm
• Decreased blood pressure
• Increased respiratory rate

Pacemakers are unaffected by common household appliances. Arc welding or powerful magnets (including those used in magnetic resonance imaging) can affect pacemaker function.

A discharging pacemaker is visible on a monitor or ECG strip. The electrical stimulus causes a *spike* or pacemaker artifact, followed by depolarization. If no pacer spike is observed and the rhythm is not dangerous, it may be that the patient's own rhythm is being sensed, and stimulation is unnecessary. However, a symptomatic individual with a pacemaker should always receive continuous monitoring.

Single-chamber pacemakers sense and pace in either the right ventricle or the right atrium.

Pacer spike   QRS

TAKE HOME POINTS

Look at the **individual**. How is the rhythm being tolerated?

- **Rate:** Because parameters are set during programming, a very fast or slow rhythm may indicate a malfunctioning pacemaker.
- **Rhythm:** Rhythm is regular, if the pacemaker is functioning appropriately.
- **P waves:** P waves are present if an atrium is being paced; they are not present if only a ventricle is being paced.
- **QRS complex:** Indicates ventricular depolarization; it should be regular in response to pacemaker stimuli. A wide QRS complex is a normal finding in paced rhythms.
- **QT interval:** It is within normal limits.

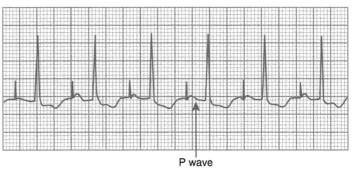

P wave

Atrial pacing.

Dual-chamber pacemakers sense and pace both the right atrium and the right ventricle in a precisely timed pattern.

Pacemakers are sophisticated, programmable devices that are designed to compensate for a failing electrical conduction system in the heart. They cannot compensate for failing heart muscle or structural damage.

Evidence of pacemaker function is visible on ECG and vital sign monitoring (pacemaker *spike* followed by evidence of depolarization).

Atrial pace spike   P wave   Ventricular pace spike   QRS

Capture occurs when an electrical stimulus has successfully depolarized the heart muscle, producing either a P wave or a QRS on ECG, depending in which chamber is electrically stimulated.

Follow ACLS guidelines when treating the individual who has a life-threatening rhythm.

What You DO

When treating patients with pacemakers, you should perform the following:
- Assess airway, breathing, circulation (ABCs).
- Continually monitor the symptomatic individual with a pacemaker. Assess the patient for pacing and capture of the pacemaker.
- Observe, document, and report changes in vital signs.
- Assess for chest pain, indigestion, changes in level of consciousness.
- Assess heart and lung sounds.
- Make available a pacemaker magnet in acute care situations. Although magnet mode varies from manufacturer to manufacturer, the magnet may be needed to temporarily disrupt pacemaker function.
- Assess for swelling of feet and ankles, jugular vein distention, and pulmonary edema.
- Teach patients to carry pacemaker identification cards and to become familiar with the settings and capabilities of implanted pacemakers.

Do You UNDERSTAND?

DIRECTIONS: **Fill in the blanks.**

1. Heart muscle contracts in response to _____ stimuli.
2. Temporary pacemakers are used in cases of _____ and _____.
3. Leads that are placed directly into the cardiac muscle through an opening in the chest are called _____ leads.
4. Leads that are placed on the inner heart wall after being threaded through a large vein via a central line are called _____ leads.
5. Most modern pacemakers can be reprogrammed using _____ and do not require additional surgery.
6. Common household appliances are safe for use by individuals with pacemakers. Powerful _____ and _____ can affect pacemaker function.
7. The pacemaker artifact seen on an ECG is called a _____.
8. _____ pacemakers sense and pace in both the right atrium and the right ventricle.
9. Pacemakers are designed to compensate for a failing electrical conduction system in the heart. They cannot compensate for _____ or _____.
10. Symptoms of pacemaker failure may include:

    _____

    _____

    _____

    _____

    _____

    _____

Answers: **1.** electrical; **2.** emergency, short-term therapy situations; **3.** epicardial; **4.** transvenous; **5.** radio frequency; **6.** magnets, arc welding; **7.** spike; **8.** Dual chamber; **9.** failing heart muscle, structural damage; **10.** Dizziness, syncope, change in mental status, difficulty breathing, weakness and fatigue, prolonged hiccups.

DRUG ABUSE

What ARE the Effects of Drug Abuse on the Heart?

The heart can be affected by the overuse and abuse of authorized and illicit drugs. These drugs include alcohol, cocaine, amphetamines, phencyclidine (PCP), inhalants, caffeine, and anabolic steroids. Some substances of abuse do not cause cardiac effects that will affect the conduction system beyond tachycardia or bradycardia. These drugs include marijuana, sedative hypnotics, opioids, and tricyclic antidepressants. They affect the central nervous system and do not usually cause dysrhythmias. However, other drugs, such as cocaine, heroin, and PCP, as well as caffeine, can produce profound and long-term effects.

What You NEED TO KNOW

Many people abuse drugs, and some die after just one episode of substance abuse. Drug abuse can affect the cardiac, pulmonary, central nervous, and metabolic systems. Drug abusers may seek health care only for an event that they perceive to be a major threat to life. Thorough assessments during routine health care check-ups can help identify patients at risk for experimentation with illicit drugs. Assessments should include ECG analysis and further questioning about current or past substance abuse.

Acute crises may require immediate stabilization with cardiac drugs, depending on the dysrhythmia or situation. Long-term drug abuse can result in chronic cardiac problems, including cardiomyopathy, congestive heart failure, and conduction problems. Many substance abusers develop significant cognitive problems from their abuse that impairs their understanding of their condition and compliance with the necessary life-style changes and medications.

TAKE HOME POINTS
- Assessment should include ECG analysis and further questioning about current or past substance abuse.
- Substance abuse can have short- and long-term cardiac consequences, depending on the substances abused.

Cocaine and Crack

Cocaine stimulates the sympathetic nervous system and is a powerful euphoric. Catecholamine (epinephrine, norepinephrine) production is increased, which elevates the heart rate by directly stimulating the SA node and atrial and ventricular tissue. Effects of cocaine and crack can be dose-related and include the following:

- Increased heart rate
- Increased force of contraction of the heart
- Increased systolic blood pressure (BP)
- Peripheral vasoconstriction, causing abdominal pain
- Atrial and ventricular dysrhythmias, including sinus tachycardia, paroxysmal supraventricular tachycardia (PSVT), atrial fibrillation and flutter, ventricular tachycardia (VT) and fibrillation, and asystole
- Increased afterload and myocardial oxygen consumption, which can lead to ischemia
- Prolongation of QT interval and QRS complex on the ECG

Coronary vasospasm, vasoconstriction, and focal endothelial damage may occur, which may increase platelet aggregation and potentiate thrombus formation. Acute myocardial infarction and cardiopulmonary arrest may occur, with or without a previous history of heart disease. Chronic, long-term cocaine abusers will develop myocarditis, pulmonary hemorrhage, and cardiomyopathy.

TAKE HOME POINTS

Afterload is the pressure against which the ventricle ejects blood.

Alcohol

Alcohol is a central nervous system depressant that causes weakness of the heart muscle and increases cardiac failure and the risk for developing pneumonia. Cardiac changes seen with chronic abuse may include cardiomyopathy. ECG changes can be seen in the QRS complex, with the entire complex being slightly wider, upright complexes being taller, and negative complexes being more negative.

Amphetamines

Amphetamines are stimulants that enhance the release of neurotransmitters. ß-adrenergic stimulation causes arterial and venous vasoconstriction. ß-adrenergic stimulation produces increases in afterload, systemic vascular response, heart rate, and contractility, greatly increasing myocardial oxygen consumption. Myocardial ischemia and infarction are major concerns as vasospasm and platelet aggregation occur. Atrial and ventricular dysrhythmias also occur.

Chronic amphetamine abuse can cause hypertension, congestive heart failure, cerebral and cardiac vasculitis with microaneurysms, and cardiomyopathy.

Phencyclidine

PCP (**angel dust, supergrass, ozone, wack, rocket fuel**) primarily affects the central nervous system, causing agitation, rage, delusions, and irrational behavior. It can cause hypertension and, in crisis stage, it can cause hypotension, bradycardia, decreased respirations, vomiting, drooling, dizziness, memory loss, and speech difficulties. PCP can be snorted, smoked (usually mixed with mint, parsley, or oregano), or eaten.

Inhalants

Many other substances, such as crack cocaine, heroin, and methamphetamines (ice) are inhaled by abusers. Their effects are primarily seen on the central nervous and pulmonary systems (heroin exacerbates asthma, which can lead to death). These effects vary with the particular chemicals being abused. The death rate from inhalant abuse may be higher than recorded, because of direct or indirect cardiotoxicity. Patients are found in VT, leading to VF and cardiac arrest, or they are found in a state of arrest when brought to the emergency department for treatment.

Caffeine

Many people would be upset to be categorized as caffeine abusers. Caffeine has a half-life of 5 hours and is a common ingredient in products containing chocolate, and in tea, soft drinks, and coffee. It is also found in some over-the-counter analgesics and herbal diuretics. Cardiac effects are dose-related and can include VT and atrial fibrillation. Few people show a bradycardic response to caffeine. Caffeine also raises BP and increases serum cholesterol. Thus caffeine increases risk for cardiovascular disease, particularly coronary heart disease.

Anabolic Steroids

Moderate to long-term use of anabolic steroids results in cardiac muscle and lipid metabolism changes. Anabolic steroids affect protein synthesis at the genetic level by affecting messenger RNA (**mRNA**) function. This alteration causes muscle cells, including cardiac cells, to hypertrophy and increase in both size and number (**hyperplastic**). This growth can result in cardiomegaly or left ventricular hypertrophy, resulting in decreased cardiac output. The effect of anabolic steroids on the lipid system is an

TAKE HOME POINTS

Acute crises may require immediate stabilization with cardiac drugs, depending on the dysrhythmia or situation.

LIFE SPAN

People who abuse drugs are found in all ages and socioeconomic groups. It is important that you carefully evaluate patients with cardiac symptoms for drug abuse, even if they have no history of heart disease.

increase in total cholesterol levels with a rising of low-density lipoproteins (LDLs) and a lowering of high-density lipoprotein (HDL) levels potentiating atherosclerotic heart disease. Often results can be reversed if the steroids are discontinued.

What You DO

When treating patients who could be abusing drugs, you should do the following:

- Assess life-style and environment frequently.
- Monitor vital signs.
- Observe ECG changes.
- Support body systems.
- Treat identified dysrhythmias.
- Monitor pH of atrial blood gases (ABGs) for acidosis.
- Monitor total serum cholesterol, LDL, and HDL levels.
- Monitor for metabolic acidosis, and prepare to give intravenous (IV) bicarbonate.
- Assess for changes in behavior, cognition, and level of consciousness.
- Assess for pulmonary hemorrhage (black sputum) and auscultate to detect increases in asthma symptoms.

Do You UNDERSTAND?

DIRECTIONS: **Fill in the blanks.**

1. Substance abusers can have the following types of acute cardiac problems:

   _____

   _____

   _____

   _____

2. Chronic substance abusers can have the following cardiac problems:

_____

_____

_____

SURGICAL THERAPY

Future challenges for effective treatment of coronary artery disease (CAD) and cardiomyopathy rests within cardiothoracic and heart transplantation surgical procedures. As a nurse, you must be able to differentiate between normal ECG changes caused by surgical approach and postoperative dysrhythmias. This section will present key points to remember in caring for patients after coronary artery bypass grafting, partial left ventriculectomy, and heart transplantation surgeries.

These surgical approaches to treat heart disease may directly affect the normal cardiac conduction system.

What IS Coronary Artery Bypass Grafting?

Coronary artery bypass grafting (CABG) (**aortocoronary bypass grafting**) is a form of surgical revascularization. This procedure bypasses coronary obstruction lesions or stenosis to restore the blood supply and flow to myocardial tissue. The procedure entails a harvested vessel or conduit (most commonly, the saphenous vein, or internal mammary artery) being anastomosed between the aortic root (base) and a distal point to the obstruction.

CABG may be indicated for the following conditions:
- Chronic stable angina pectoris
- Significant left main coronary artery occlusion (greater than 60%)
- Unstable angina with multivessel disease

- Acute MI
- Symptoms of ischemic or impending MI
- Reocclusion after percutaneous transluminal coronary angioplasty (PTCA)
- Left ventricular failure
- Intractable ventricular irritability

What You NEED TO KNOW

Intracellular myocardial edema, surgical manipulation, premature rewarming disruption of normal coronary perfusion, metabolic and electrolyte imbalances, atrial irritability, increased sympathetic stimulation, hypoxemia, hypotension, and other factors can cause injury to the cardiac conduction system. The cardiac dysrhythmias caused by these factors include the following:

- Tachydysrhythmias
- Premature ventricular contractions (PVCs)
- Bradydysrhythmias
- VT, which can occur in the immediate postoperative period

Each of these dysrhythmias must be observed and treated immediately to prevent further injury to the patient. Some dysrhythmias, such as PVCs, usually occur on the second to third postoperative day. Treatment for the dysrhythmia is aimed at preventing adverse hemodynamic effects, setting the stage for a decrease in cardiac output.

If hypoxemia and metabolic imbalances are ruled out, pharmacologic management is warranted. Depending on the dysrhythmia, drug therapy may include amiodarone, ß-blockers, class I antidysrhythmics, and calcium channel blockers.

The most common dysrhythmias reported after CABG are atrial fibrillation and atrial flutter.

Bradydysrhythmias can be caused by injury to the conduction system during surgery. Bundle branch block (BBB) or a complete AV block may be observed. The most common treatment is the use of a temporary or dual-chamber pacing device.

Atrial Dysrhythmias

ECG Findings in Atrial Fibrillation:

Redrawn from Cohn, Gilroy-Doohan: *Flip and see ECG,* Philadelphia, 1996, Saunders, p. 85.

- **Rate:** Variable according to ventricular response (less than 100 bpm—controlled atrial fibrillation; more than 100 bpm—uncontrolled atrial fibrillation)
- **Rhythm:** Irregularly irregular
- **P wave:** No true P waves (may vary from course to fine)
- **PR interval:** Not measurable
- **QRS complex:** Usually normal; may be aberrant
- **QT interval:** Not measurable

Ventricular dysrhythmias may be life-threatening. Treatment must occur immediately and is aimed at restoring adequate tissue perfusion.

ECG Findings in Atrial Flutter:

Redrawn from Cohn, Gilroy-Doohan: *Flip and see ECG,* Philadelphia, 1996, Saunders, p. 83.

- **Rates:** Atrial—250 to 400 bpm; ventricular—variable, depending on degree of AV block
- **Rhythm:** Atrial—regular; ventricular—regular or irregular
- **P wave:** "Saw tooth" flutter waves

TAKE HOME POINTS

To determine the ECG adverse effects postoperatively, observe for major dysrhythmias.

- **PR interval:** Not measurable
- **QRS complex:** Normal (0.04 to 0.11 seconds); unchanged conduction beyond the AV node
- **QT interval:** Not measurable

What You DO

When treating patients who have just undergone CABG, you should do the following:
- Continuously monitor the ECG.
- Observe for the onset of dysrhythmias (especially atrial fibrillation and VT).
- Notify the primary health care provider as soon as you notice any dysrhythmia.
- Monitor BP, level of consciousness, and peripheral perfusion.
- Prepare for cardioversion as directed by the primary health care provider.
- Administer prescribed medications, such as α-blockers, class I antidysrhythmics, and calcium channel blockers.
- Monitor effects of treatment.

Do You UNDERSTAND?

DIRECTIONS: **Fill in the blanks.**
1. List five causes of potential injury to the cardiac conduction system after CABG:

   _____

   _____

   _____

   _____

   _____

2. Most common dysrhythmias reported after CABG are
   _____ and _____ caused by
   increased _____.

Answers: 1. Intracellular myocardial edema, surgical manipulation, premature rewarming, metabolic imbalances, disruption of normal coronary perfusion; 2. atrial flutter, atrial fibrillation, atrial irritability.

What IS Cardiac Transplantation?

Cardiac transplantation is a surgical procedure that removes and replaces the diseased heart. The most common procedure is orthotopic transplantation, in which the posterior walls of the patient's atria remain and the rest of the diseased heart is removed. The remaining posterior atria walls are used to anchor the donor heart in place.

After the patient is placed on cardiopulmonary bypass, the heart is removed.

The posterior walls of the patient's left and right atria are left intact.

The left atrium of the donor heart is anastomosed to the patient's residual posterior atrial walls, and the other atrial walls, atrial septum, and great vessels are joined.

Postoperative result.

What You NEED TO KNOW

The recipient's SA node remains intact. Impulses may be initiated, but they do not cross the suture line. This causes nonconducted P waves to be observed on the ECG. The SA node of the donor's heart produces the electrical impulse that results in a cardiac contraction. Therefore a finding unique to heart transplant patients is a second P wave on ECG.

- The patient cannot tolerate intense exercise or strenuous activity. Orthostatic hypotension has been observed in patients postoperatively.
- The patient will exhibit ineffective responses to certain drugs (atropine or digitalis) or carotid sinus pressure.

TAKE HOME POINTS

To determine ECG changes for patients having undergone cardiac transplantation, you should observe for the following:

- **Rate:** Resting heart rate is between 90 and 100 bpm; there is slow or no response with an increase in heart rate caused by sympathetic stimulation.
- **Rhythm:** Donor rhythm is regular; donor P waves produce a consistent PR interval.
- **P waves:** Two P waves are visible.
- **PR interval:** Donor P waves are uniform and present before each QRS complex. Recipient P waves cause an unrelated, independent atrial rate with no direct effect on cardiac contraction.
- **QRS complex:** Complexes are normal in appearance, with a width of 0.04 to 0.10 seconds unless right BBB has developed. If an immunosuppressive drug (cyclosporin) is used, the voltage of the QRS complex may be decreased.
- **QT interval:** Intervals are measurable within normal limits unless right BBB has developed.

⚠️ Because of myocardial edema, sinus bradycardia may be observed. Isoproterenol may be used. Atrial dysrhythmias may been evident for up to 6 months postoperatively.

In addition, a right BBB is common postoperatively, because of the disruption of normal innervation of the conduction system. Denervation (absence of autonomic innervation) effects on the transplanted heart include the following:

- Lack of responsiveness to vagal stimulation, causing the patient to have a resting heart rate of 90 to 110 bpm
- Slow or no response (increased heart rate, contractility, decreased cardiac output) to sympathetic stimulation (exercise or stress)
- Dependency on circulating catecholamines and an increased venous return for the management of heart rate and contractility
- Lack of anginal chest pain with recurrent CAD. Cardiac catheterization is the only diagnostic tool to evaluate recurrence of CAD.

What You DO

When treating the patient who has just undergone cardiac transplantation, you should remember to perform the following:

- Continuously monitor the ECG for atrial and ventricular dysrhythmias.
- Observe for SVT. Treatment for this dysrhythmia is limited because of denervation of the heart. Vagal maneuvers will have no effect on heart rate. Cardioversion may be required.
- Ventricular dysrhythmias may occur. Observe for the onset of premature ventricular contractions.
- Monitor vital signs and cardiac output.
- Notify health care provider of dysrhythmias.
- Monitor for neurologic complications such as cerebrovascular accident, seizures, and headache.

Do You UNDERSTAND?

DIRECTIONS: **Fill in the blanks.**

1. The major cause for conduction changes postcardiac transplantation is

    _____.

2. What diagnostic test is used to evaluate the recurrence of CAD?

    _____.

Answers: **1. denervation, which causes an absence of autonomic innervation effect on the transplanted heart; 2. Cardiac catheterization.**

CARDIAC TRAUMA

Are you ready to meet the challenge of cardiac trauma? Knowledge, skills, and experience with ECGs may mean the difference between life and death for your patients. Examples of cardiac trauma are cardiac contusions, penetrating wounds, and cardiac tamponade.

What IS a Cardiac Trauma?

Cardiac Contusion

Cardiac contusion is soft-tissue trauma caused by a blow or blunt force to the chest. Symptoms indicating cardiac contusion include the following:
* Ecchymosis on chest wall
* Pericardial friction rub
* Tachycardia (see Chapter 9)
* Retrosternal angina that is unrelieved by nitroglycerin

Penetrating Wound

A penetrating wound is caused by an object piercing the heart. The heart may be penetrated either from the abdomen or back. Symptoms indicating penetrating wounds include the following:
* Bleeding
* Chest pain
* Loss of consciousness
* Agitation
* Muffled heart sounds
* Hypotension
* Distended neck veins
* Tachycardia
* ECG readings indicating cardiac arrest

Cardiac Tamponade

Cardiac tamponade is caused by fluid, blood, or blood clots that accumulate in the pericardial space. As fluid volume increases around the heart chambers, they are unable to completely fill with blood, and cardiac output significantly decreases or stops. Tamponade occurs as the result of cardiac contusions, penetrating wounds, recent cardiac surgery, infectious pericardial neoplasm, or uremia (see Chapter 20). In addition, it may be a complication following pericardial taps, cardiac catheterization, cardiopulmonary resuscitation (CPR), or pacemaker insertion. Symptoms of cardiac tamponade include the following:

- Decreased cardiac output
- Pulsus paradoxus (decrease in systolic BP of greater than 10 mm Hg during inspiration if monitoring with an arterial line; or a palpable decrease in pulse during inspiration)
- Muffled heart sounds
- Jugular venous distention with clear lungs
- Hypotension
- Increased central venous pressure
- Narrowed pulse pressure

Pulse pressure is measured by subtracting the diastolic BP from the systolic BP. If the BP is 120/80 mm Hg, you would subtract 80 from 120 to get a pulse pressure of 40 (120 − 80 = 40). It is normally one third of the systolic BP. Pulse pressure narrows (gets smaller) in cardiac tamponade as pressures in the heart equalize.

The following ECG changes may be seen in cardiac trauma. They mimic myocardial injury, ischemia, or infarction:

- ST segment elevation
- T wave changes (tall T waves)
- Possibility of deep or wide Q waves
- Diminished ECG amplitude

Redrawn from Ignatavicius, Workman, Mishler: *Medical-surgical nursing across the health care continuum,* ed 2, Philadelphia, 1995, Saunders, p. 835.

What You NEED TO KNOW

You should consider any patient with cardiac trauma to be an emergency; immediate action is required. Continuous ECG monitoring is imperative.

What You DO

When treating the patient in cardiac trauma, you should perform the following:
- Consider the situation an emergency, and act quickly.
- Assess the ABCs.
- Notify the primary health care provider of any dysrhythmias.
- Continuously monitor the ECG.
- Monitor closely for shock.
- Begin IV therapy.
- Draw blood for laboratory type and cross matching.
- Get complete medical history.
- Administer oxygen.
- Assist the primary health care provider with insertion of chest tube or pericardiocentesis.
- Prepare for possible thoracotomy.

TAKE HOME POINTS
To determine ECG changes in a patient with cardiac trauma, you should observe for the following:
- **Rate:** Rapid
- **Rhythm:** Dysrhythmic, diminished amplitude
- **QRS complex:** Tall T waves; possible deep or wide Q waves

Do You UNDERSTAND?

DIRECTIONS: **Fill in the blanks.**
1. List three examples of cardiac trauma.

_____

_____

_____

Answers: **1. cardiac contusion, penetrating wound, cardiac tamponade.**

2. ECG changes with cardiac trauma mimic the following conditions:

_____

_____

_____

DIRECTIONS: **Indicate in the spaces provided whether the following statements are *true* or *false*.**

3. _____ Dysrhythmias are common in cardiac trauma.

4. _____ Cardiac tamponade is a result of a myocardial infarction.

5. _____ Suspect cardiac tamponade when ECG changes indicate a tall T wave, diminished amplitude, and ST segment elevation.

References

AHA Scientific Position: *Sudden cardiac death*. Available online at www.americanheart.org/presenter.jhtml?identifier=4741.

Borer A et al: Prevention of infections associated with permanent cardiac antiarrythmic devices by implementation of a comprehensive infection control program, *Infect Control Hosp Epidemiol* 25(6):492-497, 2004.

Gambino A: Challenges of heart transplantation: now and the future, *Transplant Proc* 35(8):3069-3071, 2003.

Ganz L: Implantable cardioverter/defibrillators, *Emedicine*, Oct 28, 2004. Available online at www.emedicine.com/med/topic3386.htm.

Malineni KC: Sudden cardiac death, *Emedicine*, Nov 11, 2004. Available online at www.emedicine.com/med/topic276.htm.

McCance K, Huether SE: *Pathophysiology: the biologic basis for disease in adults and children*, ed 4, St Louis, 2002, Mosby.

Thelan LA et al: *Critical care nursing: diagnosis and management,* ed 4, St Louis, 2002, Mosby.

NCLEX® Review

1. A patient who is known to have an internal cardioverter-defibrillator (ICD) is admitted to the cardiac care unit with intermittent episodes of dizziness and palpitations. Which of the following should the health care provider do first?
   1 Deactivate the ICD by placing a pacemaker magnet over the pulse generator.
   2 Obtain a 12-lead ECG.
   3 Ensure that resuscitation equipment is available, and monitor the patient's rhythm continuously.
   4 Teach the patient relaxation techniques and deep breathing.

2. A patient who has recently had an ICD implanted is learning about the device. Which of the following statements by the patient demonstrates an understanding of the purpose of this device?
   1 The ICD uses electrical impulses to control dangerous heart rhythms.
   2 The ICD will prevent dangerous heart rhythms from occurring.
   3 The ICD will make my heart stronger.
   4 The ICD will prevent my heart beat from slowing down too much.

3. A patient who has had an ICD implanted expresses anxiety regarding the sensation that will be felt when the device discharges. Appropriate teaching on the part of the health care provider includes which of the following statements?
   1 "When the device discharges, it will make you faint."
   2 "When the device discharges, you will not even feel it."
   3 "Different patients experience the discharging of the device in different ways."
   4 "Different patients have different pain thresholds, but it shouldn't bother you too much."

4. A patient is admitted to the hospital unit following a transvenous pacemaker placement. The patient denies pain but is uncomfortable because of unrelenting hiccups. Vital signs are within normal limits, and respirations are unlabored. An appropriate action on the part of the health care provider is to:
   1 Ascertain that the patient has an intact gag reflex, then offer clear liquids
   2 Determine how the patient treats hiccups at home, and assist in carrying out the treatment
   3 Call the physician to report the hiccups, and place the patient on continuous cardiac monitoring
   4 Position the patient on the right side, and contact the physician for a chlorpromazine (Thorazine) order

5. Which of the following patient statements indicates an understanding of pacemaker precautions?
   1 "I should avoid microwave ovens."
   2 "I should avoid high frequency sounds."
   3 "I should avoid cordless telephones."
   4 "I should avoid powerful magnetic sources."

6. Reprogramming of implanted permanent pacemakers is accomplished by:
   1 A simple outpatient surgical procedure
   2 Radio frequencies transmitted through the skin
   3 A pacemaker magnet
   4 A telephone call to the health care provider's office

7. Mrs. Flanceski is a patient admitted to the ambulatory surgery unit for a minor orthopedic procedure. The patient states she is feeling well this morning. Her chart indicates that she has an implanted dual-chamber pacemaker. When the nurse initiates ECG monitoring per unit procedure, the patient's heart rate is 80 bpm but no pacemaker spikes are visible. This situation indicates that:
   1 Mrs. Flanceski needs a battery replacement for her pacemaker
   2 Mrs. Flanceski needs her pacemaker reprogrammed
   3 The physician should be notified and resuscitation equipment taken to the bedside
   4 The pacemaker is sensing Mrs. Flanceski's naturally occurring heart rate

8. Cardiomyopathy is a common cardiac problem for individuals who chronically abuse drugs. Which of the following drugs would not cause this problem?
   1 Cocaine
   2 Marijuana
   3 Amphetamines
   4 Alcohol

9. Myocardial infarction can occur with use of which of the following illicit drugs?
   1 Alcohol
   2 Crack
   3 Angel dust
   4 All of the above

10. Mr. Smith underwent a cardiac transplantation 24 hours ago. The health care provider observed a change in his ECG strip that indicated a supraventricular tachycardia. The treatment of choice is:
    1 Digitalis
    2 Carotid sinus pressure
    3 Cardioversion
    4 Valsalva maneuver

11. As an emergency nurse, you have just received a patient who had been in a motorcycle accident. It was reported that the motorcycle had landed on his chest. Ecchymotic lesions were evident on the chest, a pericardial friction rub was heard, and retrosternal pain was present. Your first priority as an emergency room nurse would be to:
    1 Obtain a complete medical history
    2 Administer oxygen
    3 Monitor the ECG
    4 Assess airway, breathing, and circulation

12. ECG changes with cardiac trauma include:
    1 Bradycardia
    2 Tachycardia
    3 Normal sinus rhythm
    4 Right bundle branch block

NCLEX® Review Answers

1. 3 The patient's symptoms may indicate a malfunctioning ICD. Resuscitation equipment should be immediately available, and the heart rhythm should be continuously monitored. The pulse generator should not be deactivated except during resuscitation. Although a 12-lead ECG would be helpful in diagnosis, it is not the first action the provider should take. Relaxation has no effect on internal defibrillation.

2. 1 The ICD controls dangerous heart rhythms. The ICD does not prevent dangerous heart rhythms from occurring or affect the strength or contractility of the heart muscle.

3. 3 Some patients experience collapse, and others are not even aware the device has discharged. Patient response to discharging of the device is an individual phenomenon. Some patients experience unconsciousness. By telling the patient that it should not "bother" him or her too much, the provider implies that if the discharge of the device is perceived to be uncomfortable, the patient must have a low pain tolerance.

4. 3 The pacemaker leads can become dislodged, irritate the diaphragm, and cause the patient to have hiccups. When pacemaker malfunction is suspected, the patient should be monitored continuously. Home remedies will not stop hiccups that are the result of a pacemaker malfunction. Putting the patient on continuous cardiac monitoring could cause more damage to the pacemaker. Although chlorpromazine (Thorazine) is sometimes used to stop hiccups, in this case it can cause more cardiac problems.

5. 4 Powerful magnetic sources may affect pacemaker function. Pacemakers are not affected by the microwave ovens in use today. Although pacemakers can be reprogrammed by radiofrequency through the skin, hearing high frequency sounds has no effect. Cordless telephones do not affect pacemaker function.

6. 2 Reprogramming of implanted permanent pacemakers is accomplished by radio frequencies transmitted through the skin. A simple surgical procedure is sometimes necessary to change the battery. A pacemaker magnet will deactivate the device. Although pacemaker function can be monitored via telephone, reprogramming cannot currently be accomplished in this way.

7. 4 Because the rate is 80 bpm, and the patient is asymptomatic, the absence of pacemaker spikes is an indication that the pacemaker is not in control of the patient's heart rhythm. Because the patient's heart rate is 80 bpm without pacing, and she is asymptomatic, it is likely that the device senses the adequacy of the patient's naturally occurring rhythm. There is no "demand" for pacing in this situation.

8. 2 Marijuana does not cause cardiomyopathy. Cocaine, amphetamines, and alcohol increase heart rate.

9. 2 Cocaine and crack use stimulates the sympathetic nervous system, increasing production of epinephrine and norepinephrine; this may cause coronary vasospasm and vasoconstriction. Local damage to the endothelial lining of the coronary vessels can cause platelet aggregation and thrombus formation. A myocardial infarction can occur with no history of heart disease. The two remaining drugs do not affect the heart in the same way. With alcohol and angel dust, no myocardial infarction occurs.

10. 3 Treatment of supraventricular tachycardia is limited because of denervation of the heart; therefore cardioversion may be required. Because of the denervation (absence of autonomic innervation) effect on the transplanted heart's responses to digitalis, carotid sinus pressure will not be effective. The Valsalva maneuver stimulates the vagus nerve, causing a slowing of the heart in a normal autonomic innervation. Because the transplanted heart is denervated, the heart is dependent upon circulating catecholamines and an increased venous return to manage heart rate and contractility.

11. 4 Maintaining the airway, breathing, and circulation is obviously essential to the life of the patient. Obtaining a complete medical history is not the first priority, and assessment is needed before treating the patient by administering oxygen. An ECG cannot provide all necessary data on the airway, breathing, and circulation.

12. 2 Tachycardia acts to increase the amount of oxygen delivered to cells of the body by increasing the amount of blood circulated through the vessels. Tachycardia accompanies anoxia, such as that caused by cardiac trauma. Only tachycardia has an increased heart rate over 100 bpm. A normal sinus rhythm is not a threat, and right bundle branch block is not associated with cardiac trauma.

Rhythm Strip Test

Strip 1 Rate: _____ Rhythm: _____ P wave: _____

    PR interval: _____ QRS: _____

    Rhythm interpretation: _____

Strip 2 Rate: _____ Rhythm: _____ P wave: _____

    PR interval: _____ QRS: _____

    Rhythm interpretation: _____

Strip 3   Rate: _____   Rhythm: _____   P wave: _____

PR interval: _____   QRS: _____

Rhythm interpretation: _____

Strip 4   Rate: _____   Rhythm: _____   P wave: _____

PR interval: _____   QRS: _____

Rhythm interpretation: _____

Strip 5   Rate: _____   Rhythm: _____   P wave: _____

PR interval: _____   QRS: _____

Rhythm interpretation: _____

Strip 6   Rate: _____   Rhythm: _____   P wave: _____

PR interval: _____   QRS: _____

Rhythm interpretation: _____

Strip 7   Rate: _____   Rhythm: _____   P wave: _____

PR interval: _____   QRS: _____

Rhythm interpretation: _____

Strip 8   Rate: _____   Rhythm: _____   P wave: _____

PR interval: _____   QRS: _____

Rhythm interpretation: _____

Strip 9   Rate: _____   Rhythm: _____   P wave: _____

PR interval: _____   QRS: _____

Rhythm interpretation: _____

Strip 10   Rate: _____   Rhythm: _____   P wave: _____

PR interval: _____   QRS: _____

Rhythm interpretation: _____

Strip 11   Rate: _____   Rhythm: _____   P wave: _____

PR interval: _____   QRS: _____

Rhythm interpretation: _____

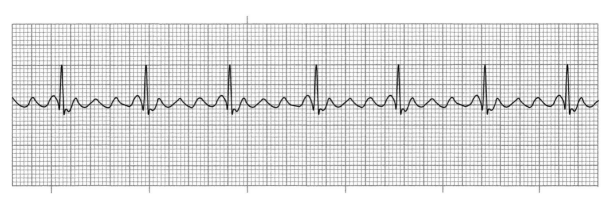

Strip 12   Rate: _____   Rhythm: _____   P wave: _____

PR interval: _____   QRS: _____

Rhythm interpretation: _____

Strip 13   Rate: _____   Rhythm: _____   P wave: _____

PR interval: _____   QRS: _____

Rhythm interpretation: _____

Strip 14   Rate: _____   Rhythm: _____   P wave: _____

PR interval: _____   QRS: _____

Rhythm interpretation: _____

Strip 15   Rate: _____   Rhythm: _____   P wave: _____

PR interval: _____   QRS: _____

Rhythm interpretation: _____

Strip 16   Rate: _____   Rhythm: _____   P wave: _____

PR interval: _____   QRS: _____

Rhythm interpretation: _____

Strip 17   Rate: _____   Rhythm: _____   P wave: _____

PR interval: _____   QRS: _____

Rhythm interpretation: _____

Strip 18   Rate: _____   Rhythm: _____   P wave: _____

PR interval: _____   QRS: _____

Rhythm interpretation: _____

Strip 19   Rate: _____   Rhythm: _____   P wave: _____

PR interval: _____   QRS: _____

Rhythm interpretation: _____

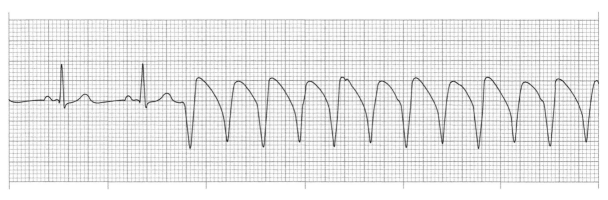

Strip 20   Rate: _____   Rhythm: _____   P wave: _____

PR interval: _____   QRS: _____

Rhythm interpretation: _____

Strip 21   Rate: _____   Rhythm: _____   P wave: _____

PR interval: _____   QRS: _____

Rhythm interpretation: _____

Strip 22   Rate: _____   Rhythm: _____   P wave: _____

PR interval: _____   QRS: _____

Rhythm interpretation: _____

Strip 23   Rate: _____   Rhythm: _____   P wave: _____

PR interval: _____   QRS: _____

Rhythm interpretation: _____

Strip 24   Rate: _____   Rhythm: _____   P wave: _____

PR interval: _____   QRS: _____

Rhythm interpretation: _____

Strip 25   Rate: _____   Rhythm: _____   P wave: _____

PR interval: _____   QRS: _____

Rhythm interpretation: _____

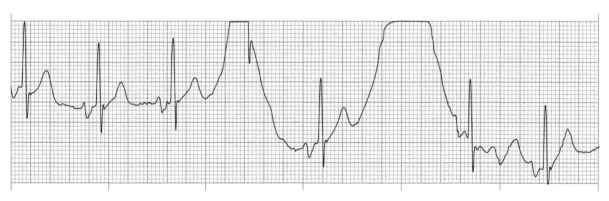

Strip 26   Rate: _____   Rhythm: _____   P wave: _____

PR interval: _____   QRS: _____

Rhythm interpretation: _____

Strip 27   Rate: _____   Rhythm: _____   P wave: _____

PR interval: _____   QRS: _____

Rhythm interpretation: _____

Strip 28   Rate: _____   Rhythm: _____   P wave: _____

PR interval: _____   QRS: _____

Rhythm interpretation: _____

Strip 29   Rate: _____   Rhythm: _____   P wave: _____

PR interval: _____   QRS: _____

Rhythm interpretation: _____

Strip 30   Rate: _____   Rhythm: _____   P wave: _____

PR interval: _____   QRS: _____

Rhythm interpretation: _____

Rhythm Strip Test Answers

Strip 1   **Rate:** 70   **Rhythm:** Regular   **P waves:** Yes
             PR interval: 0.16 seconds   **QRS:** 0.08 seconds
             Rhythm interpretation: Normal sinus rhythm

Strip 2   **Rate:** 40   **Rhythm:** Regular   **P waves:** Yes
             PR interval: 0.16 seconds   **QRS:** 0.08 seconds
             Rhythm interpretation: Sinus bradycardia

Strip 3   **Rate:** 140   **Rhythm:** Regular   **P waves:** Yes
             PR interval: 0.16 seconds   **QRS:** 0.08 seconds
             Rhythm interpretation: Sinus tachycardia

Strip 4   **Rate:** 195   **Rhythm:** Regular   **P waves:** Yes
             PR interval: 0.14-0.16 seconds   **QRS:** 0.08 seconds
             Rhythm interpretation: Atrial tachycardia (supraventricular tachycardia)

Strip 5   **Rate:** 70   **Rhythm:** Regular   **P waves:** Yes, inverted
             PR interval: N/A   **QRS:** 0.06-0.08 seconds
             Rhythm interpretation: Accelerated junctional rhythm

Strip 6   **Rate:** 70   **Rhythm:** Irregular   **P waves:** Yes, but only with
             PR interval: 0.16 seconds   **QRS:** 0.08 with normal beats   normal sinus beats
                                               (0.14 seconds with PVCs)
             Rhythm interpretation: Ventricular bigeminy (every other beat is a PVC)

Strip 7   **Rate:** Not measurable   **Rhythm:** Chaotic   **P waves:** No
             PR interval: N/A   **QRS:** N/A
             Rhythm interpretation: Ventricular fibrillation

Strip 8   **Rate:** 60   **Rhythm:** Irregular (groups of beats) **P waves:** Yes
             PR interval: progressively   **QRS:** 0.08 seconds
             prolongs in each group
             Rhythm interpretation: Wenckebach (Type I, second-degree heart block)

Strip 9   **Rate:** 40   **Rhythm:** Regular   **P waves:** Yes, inverted
             PR interval: N/A   **QRS:** 0.08 seconds
             Rhythm interpretation: Junctional rhythm

Strip 10 **Rate:** Atrial rate 100; 40   **Rhythm:** Regular   **P waves:** More Ps than QRS'
             ventricular rate
             PR interval: 0.16 when there is a QRS **QRS:** 0.08 seconds
             Rhythm interpretation: Type II, second-degree heart block

Strip 11 **Rate:** 70   **Rhythm:** Irregular   **P waves:** Yes
             PR interval: 0.16 seconds   **QRS:** 0.08 seconds
             Rhythm interpretation: Normal sinus rhythm with premature atrial contractions (PACs) on third and
             seventh beats

Strip 12   **Rate:** Atrial rate 300;   **Rhythm:** Regular   **P waves:** No (flutter waves)
ventricular rate 40
PR interval: Indeterminate   **QRS:** 0.08 seconds
Rhythm interpretation: Atrial flutter

Strip 13   **Rate:** 80   **Rhythm:** Irregular (second   **P waves:** Yes, upright with
PR interval: 0.16 seconds with   and fourth beats are premature)   sinus beats, inverted with
sinus beats   **QRS:** 0.08 seconds   premature beats
Rhythm interpretation: Sinus rhythm with premature junctional contractions (PJCs)

Strip 14   **Rate:** 40   **Rhythm:** Regular   **P waves:** Several P waves (more Ps
PR interval: Not consistent   **QRS:** 0.18 seconds   than QRS')
Rhythm interpretation: Third-degree AV block (complete heart block) with ventricular escape rhythm

Strip 15   **Rate:** About 100   **Rhythm:** Totally irregular   **P waves:** No
PR interval: N/A   **QRS:** 0.06 seconds
Rhythm interpretation: Atrial fibrillation

Strip 16   **Rate:** 80   **Rhythm:** Regular   **P waves:** No
PR interval: Indeterminate   **QRS:** 0.16 seconds
Rhythm interpretation: 100% paced rhythm (ventricles are being paced; spike occurs before the QRS)

Strip 17   **Rate:** 70   **Rhythm:** Regular   **P waves:** Yes
PR interval: 0.16 seconds   **QRS:** 0.08 seconds
Rhythm interpretation: Normal sinus rhythm

Strip 18   **Rate:** 80   **Rhythm:** Irregular   **P waves:** Only with sinus beats
PR interval: 0.16 seconds   **QRS:** 0.08 seconds
Rhythm interpretation: Sinus rhythm with multifocal couplets (two PVCs in a row)

Strip 19   **Rate:** 70   **Rhythm:** Irregular   **P waves:** With sinus beats
PR interval: 0.16 seconds   **QRS:** Variable
Rhythm interpretation: Sinus rhythm with unifocal PVCs

Strip 20   **Rate:** 70-160   **Rhythm:** Irregular   **P waves:** With sinus beats (first
PR interval: 0.16 seconds   **QRS:** variable   two beats)
with sinus beats
Rhythm interpretation: Two sinus beats with onset of ventricular tachycardia

Strip 21   **Rate:** None   **Rhythm:** None   **P wave:** None
PR interval: Indeterminate   **QRS:** No QRS complexes
Rhythm interpretation: Asystole

Strip 22   **Rate:** 138   **Rhythm:** Regular   **P waves:** Yes
PR interval: 0.20 seconds   **QRS:** 0.06 seconds
Rhythm interpretation: Sinus tachycardia

Strip 23   **Rate:** 42   **Rhythm:** Regular   **P waves:** Yes
                PR interval: 0.24 seconds   **QRS:** 0.06-0.08 seconds
                Rhythm interpretation: Sinus bradycardia with first-degree AV block (PRI > 0.20 seconds)

Strip 24   **Rate:** 62   **Rhythm:** Regular   **P waves:** No (flutter waves)
                PR interval: Indeterminate   **QRS:** 0.10 seconds
                Rhythm interpretation: Atrial flutter

Strip 25   **Rate:** 61   **Rhythm:** Regular   **P waves:** Yes, inverted
                PR interval: 0.16 seconds   **QRS:** 0.08 seconds
                Rhythm interpretation: Accelerated junctional rhythm

Strip 26   **Rate:** 77   **Rhythm:** Regular   **P waves:** Yes, biphasic
                PR interval: 0.16 seconds   **QRS:** 0.10 seconds
                Rhythm interpretation: Poor quality tracing; sinus rhythm with artifact

Strip 27   **Rate:** About 30   **Rhythm:** Irregular   **P waves:** No
                PR interval: N/A   **QRS:** 0.24 seconds
                Rhythm interpretation: Ventricular escape rhythm (idioventricular rhythm)

Strip 28   **Rate:** 70→170→70   **Rhythm:** Irregular   **P waves:** With sinus beats
                PR interval: 0.16 seconds   **QRS:** 0.08-0.14 seconds
                with sinus beats
                Rhythm interpretation: Sinus rhythm with a run of ventricular tachycardia

Strip 29   **Rate:** Atrial rate 300,   **Rhythm:** Slightly irregular   **P waves:** No (flutter waves)
                ventricular rate 118   **QRS:** 0.10 seconds
                PR interval: Indeterminate
                Rhythm interpretation: Atrial flutter

Strip 30   **Rate:** Indeterminate   **Rhythm:** Chaotic   **P waves:** No
                PR interval: Indeterminate   **QRS:** Indeterminate
                Rhythm interpretation: Ventricular fibrillation

Index

Page numbers followed by *t* indicate tables.

Brachiocephalic trunk

Superior vena cava

Right pulmonary
artery

Ascending aorta

Right pulmonary
veins

Right coronary artery
and cardiac vein

Right atrium

Right ventricle

Left common carotid artery

Left subclavian artery

Arch of aorta

Left pulmonary
artery

Left atrium

Left pulmonary
veins

Great cardiac
vein

Branches of left
coronary artery
and cardiac vein

Left ventricle

Apex

S

R — L

I

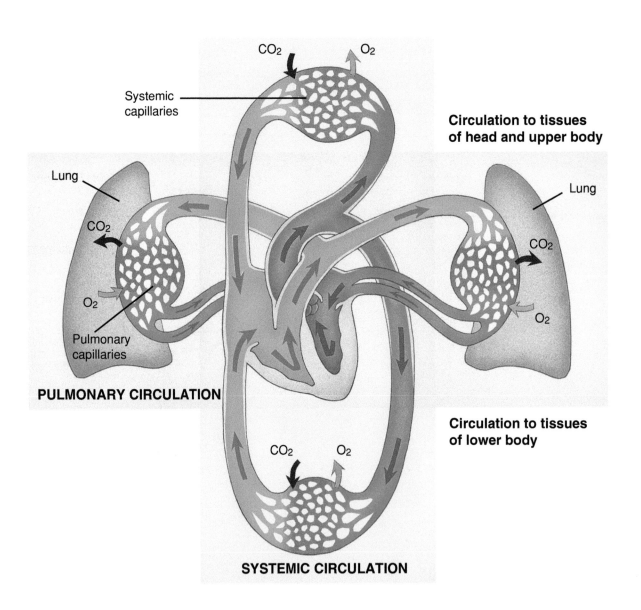

CO$_2$ O$_2$

Systemic capillaries

Circulation to tissues of head and upper body

Lung

CO$_2$

O$_2$

Pulmonary capillaries

PULMONARY CIRCULATION

Lung

CO$_2$

O$_2$

Circulation to tissues of lower body

CO$_2$ O$_2$

SYSTEMIC CIRCULATION

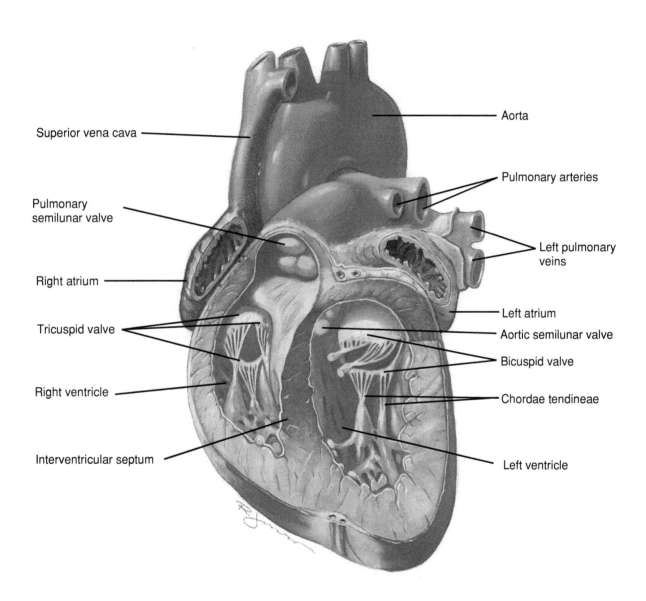

Superior vena cava

Pulmonary
semilunar valve

Right atrium

Tricuspid valve

Right ventricle

Interventricular septum

Aorta

Pulmonary arteries

Left pulmonary
veins

Left atrium

Aortic semilunar valve

Bicuspid valve

Chordae tendineae

Left ventricle

Atrial Fibrillation and Atrial Flutter Algorithm

Perform Primary ABCD Survey (Basic Life Support)
- Correct critical problems IMMEDIATELY as they are identified
- Assess responsiveness, Airway, Breathing, Circulation; ensure availability of monitor and Defibrillator

Perform Secondary ABCD Survey (Advanced Life Support)
- Administer oxygen, establish IV access, attach cardiac monitor, administer fluids as needed (O_2, IV, monitor, fluids)
- Assess vital signs, attach pulse oximeter, and monitor blood pressure
- Obtain and review 12-lead ECG and portable chest x-ray; perform a focused history and physical examination

> Is the patient stable or unstable? Is the patient experiencing serious signs and symptoms caused by tachycardia? Is the patient's cardiac function normal or impaired? Attempt to identify patient's cardiac rhythm using 12-lead ECG and clinical information. Is Wolff-Parkinson-White syndrome (WPW) present? If yes, see WPW syndrome, Chapter 22, page 341. Has atrial fibrillation or atrial flutter been present for more or less than 48 hours?

Stable Patient

Normal Cardiac Function		Impaired Cardiac Function	
Onset < 48 hours	Onset > 48 hours	Onset < 48 hours	Onset > 48 hours
Control Rate	**Control Rate**	**Control Rate**	**Control Rate**
Calcium channel blocker (Class I) OR Beta-blocker (Class I) OR Digoxin (IIb)	Calcium channel blocker (Class I) OR Beta-blocker (Class I) OR Digoxin (IIb)	Diltiazem (IIb) OR Amiodarone (IIb) OR Digoxin (IIb)	Diltiazem (IIb) OR Amiodarone (IIb) OR Digoxin (IIb)
Convert Rhythm	**Convert Rhythm**	**Convert Rhythm**	**Convert Rhythm**
Cardioversion OR Amiodarone (IIa) OR Procainamide (IIa) OR Ibutilide (IIa) OR Flecainide (IIa) OR Propafenone (IIa)	Delayed cardioversion OR Early cardioversion	Cardioversion OR Amiodarone (IIb)	Delayed cardioversion OR Early cardioversion

Delayed cardioversion: Anticoagulation therapy for 3 weeks before cardioversion for at least 48 hours in conjunction with cardioversion and for at least 4 weeks after successful cardioversion

Early cardioversion: IV heparin immediately, transesophageal echocardiography (TEE) to rule out atrial thrombus; cardioversion within 24 hours; anticoagulation for 4 weeks

Unstable Patient

If hemodynamically unstable, perform synchronized cardioversion:

Atrial fibrillation: 100, 200, 300, or 360 J, or equivalent biphasic energy

Atrial flutter: 50, 100, 200, 300, or 360 J, or equivalent biphasic energy

Medication dosing: **Amiodarone**—150 mg IV bolus over 10 minutes, followed by an infusion of 1 mg/min for 6 hours and then a maintenance infusion of 0.5 mg/min. Repeat supplementary infusions of 150 mg as necessary for recurrent or resistant dysrhythmias. Maximum total daily dose 2.2 g. **Beta blockers**—*Esmolol:* 0.5 mg/kg over 1 minute followed by a maintenance infusion at 50 µg/kg/min for 4 minutes. If inadequate response, administer a second bolus of 0.5 mg/kg over 1 minute and increase maintenance infusion to 100 µg/kg/min. The bolus dose (0.5 mg/kg) and titration of the maintenance infusion (addition of 50 µg/kg/min) can be repeated every 4 minutes to a maximum infusion of 300 µg/kg/min. *Metoprolol:* 5 mg slow IV push over 5 minutes three times as needed to a total dose of 15 mg over 15 minutes. *Propranolol:* 0.1 mg/kg slow IV push divided in three equal doses at 2 to 3 minute intervals. Do not exceed 1 mg/min. Repeat after 2 minutes if necessary. *Atenolol:* 5 mg slow IV (over 5 minutes). Wait 10 minutes; then give second dose of 5 mg slow IV (over 5 minutes). **Calcium channel blockers**—*Diltiazem:* 0.25 mg/kg over 2 minutes (e.g., 15 to 20 mg). If ineffective, 0.35 mg/kg over 2 minutes (e.g., 20 to 25 mg) in 15 minutes. Maintenance infusion 5 to 15 mg/hr, titrated to heart rate if chemical conversion is successful. Calcium chloride (2 to 4 mg/kg) may be given slow IV push if borderline hypotension exists before diltiazem administration. *Verapamil:* 2.5 to 5.0 mg slow IV push over 2 minutes. May repeat with 5 to 10 mg in 15 to 30 minutes. Maximum dose 20 mg. **Ibutilide**—Adults ≥ 60 kg: 1 mg (10 mL) over 10 minutes. May repeat once in 10 minutes. Adults < 60 kg: 0.01 mg/kg IV over 10 minutes. **Procainamide**—100 mg over 5 minutes (20 mg/min). Maximum total dose 17 mg/kg. Maintenance infusion 1 to 4 mg/min. **Flecainide, propafenone**—IV form not currently approved for use in the United States. **Sotalol**—1.0 to 1.5 mg/kg IV slowly at a rate of 10 mg/min.

Adapted from first edition of this text.